Jewish Ethics and the Care of End-of-Life Patients

A Collection of Rabbinical, Bioethical, Philosophical, and Juristic Opinions

Jewish Ethics and the Care of End-of-Life Patients

A Collection of Rabbinical, Bioethical, Philosophical, and Juristic Opinions

EDITED BY

Peter Joel Hurwitz, Jacques Picard,
and Avraham Steinberg

ARTICLES WRITTEN IN GERMAN AND HEBREW
WERE TRANSLATED BY

Dr. Benjamin Sklarz

KTAV Publishing House, Inc.
Jersey City, N.J.

in association with
The Institute for Jewish Studies, University of Basel
Basel, Switzerland

Library of Congress Cataloging-in-Publication Data

Jewish ethics and the care of end-of-life patients: a collection of rabbinical,
   bioethical, philosophical, and juristic opinions / edited by Peter Joel
   Hurwitz, Jacques Picard, and Avraham Steinberg.
      p. cm.
   Includes bibliographical references.
   ISBN 0-88125-921-7
   1. Death – Religious aspects – Judaism. 2. Terminal care – Religious
aspects – Judaism. 3. Euthanasia. 4. Terminally ill – Legal status, laws,
etc. – Israel.   I. Hurwitz, Peter Joel. II. Picard, Jacques. III. Steinberg,
Avraham.
   [DNLM: 1. Bioethical Issues. 2. Terminal Care – ethics. 3. Judaism.
4. Palliative Care – ethics. 5. Terminally Ill. 6. Religion and Medicine.
WB 60 J59 2006]
BM635.4.J384 2006
296.3>697 – dc22

                                                                    2005038053

Manufactured in the United States of America

Published by
KTAV Publishing House, Inc.
930 Newark Avenue
Jersey City, NJ 07306
Tel. (201) 963-9524
Fax. (201) 963-0102
www.ktav.com
bernie@ktav.com

Typeset by Jerusalem Typesetting, www.jerusalemtype.com
Cover Design by Oscar Rijo

Table of Contents

Preface

Jacques Picard

W E ARE LIVING in a time when the perceived borderline between life and nonlife has become uncertain, and we are made particularly aware of this when talking about birth and death. The extrauterine generation of life made possible by medicine, *in vitro* fertilization, has contributed to a shift in our views, long cherished as valid, about how and when life begins. This poses dilemmas for us in the use of stem cells, which are being exploited for basic research in the hope of achieving medical advances, and also with regard to preimplantational diagnostics, prenatal diagnostics, and interruption of pregnancy. In laboratories, and through the logic of research, the difference between biological forms of life and their simulations in the computer world is disappearing, and both realms seem to be linked. In an equally far-reaching manner, questions are arising at the end of human life. We are forced to consider new definitions of death as drugs, artificial nutrition, transplants, and technical devices allow the prolongation of life. Where does life begin, and where does it end? The borderline has become fluid.

All this has changed even our everyday thinking about death. Perhaps, after long drawn-out illness and suffering, we may accept death for ourselves or a fellow human being without resignation, after rage, rebellion, mourning, and acceptance are manifested. We may, after an initial shock, wish to regard even an accidental and surprising case of death as a matter of fate. Every time we lose a near and dear one,

1

we sense that the borderline between death and life can somehow be invisible, and we thus become unsure from which side we regard ourselves. It is as if death has always been present in our lives. But never have we faced the situation of having to decide when a failing life should end in death as it arises from the question whether or not to stop artificial nutrition or to switch off some machine. Medical advances have presented us with such questions.

This possibility as well as further echoes of our experiences are frequently called into play, particularly in the matter of prolongation of life, through the possibilities offered by contemporary medicine. Momentous considerations are faced by the dying, their relations, the doctors, and everyone else involved with life and death. Must "everything be done" to prolong life? By what means is this to be achieved? And what happens if medical procedures are unavailable for economic reasons? Can preventing a desperately ill person from dying, even against his or her will, really be the "supreme commandment"? And who may or may not decide? These questions are merely a few points from the debate currently proceeding in many countries, religions, and cultures around the world. Historical experiences also remain with us as we grapple with this theme, such as memories of the horrendous acts of the Nazis, whose political creed once made a distinction between valuable and "valueless" lives. These circumstances sharpen our awareness of the inviolability of human dignity, which, in the words of the Talmud (BT Berakhot 19b), can even override laws of the Torah.

This book contributes a Jewish viewpoint to a universal debate. More precisely it presents several Jewish perspectives, some mutually contradictory. But their very diverseness can provide us with insights in a discussion which arises out of a long-lived interpretational culture, at whose center stood and stands the relationship between man and man and between man and God. *Torah ve-hayyim* – one may not put the Torah, the Law, in opposition to life. Indeed, the search for guidance from the ways and teachings of Jewish tradition must start out from the requirements of society. This dynamic tradition can yield insights which will enrich the universal discussion and the broad human struggle concerning the ethical questions of terminal care and assisted death. Palliative medicine and practical aspects of terminal care for care-givers are also treated by the contributions here presented.

Thanks to the initiative of Peter Joel Hurwitz, this book has emerged from the cooperation of its three editors, and Abraham Steinberg, chairman of the Israel Governmental Commission on the questions addressed by this book, has agreed to serve as an additional editor. One must give cordial thanks to all the authors. Bernard Scharfstein of Ktav Publishing House has contributed to the book's publication by his spirited cooperation. I would like to list the sponsors whose contributions made possible the translations and the publication of the book: the Fund for Promotion of the Humanities of the Freiwillige Akademische Gesellschaft, Basle; the Georges and Jenny Bloch Foundation; the Irene Bollag-Herzheimer Foundation; the Käthe Zingg-Schwichtenberg Fund of the Swiss Academy for Medical Sciences (Schweizerischen Akademie der Medizinischen Wissenschaften); and the Dean's Medical Legacies Fund of the Medical Faculty and University Hospital, Basle (Medizinischer Vermächtnisfonds am Dekanat der Medizinischen Fakultät und Universitätsspital Basel). Dr. Lutz Zwillenberg of Bern has supported us with a personal financial contribution. Our thanks are hereby extended to all of them. We should also mention that the Institute for Jewish Studies at the University of Basle donated space for the creation of this book. We are furthermore obliged to our colleagues Alfred Bodenheimer and Ekkehard Stegemann. I wish to announce the simultaneous publication of a German-language edition of this book by Schwabe Verlag in Basle.

On a personal note, my mother, Ida Picard-Rawyler, passed away peacefully after a long and full life while this book was in the process of preparation: I cherish her memory.

Institute for Jewish Studies
University of Basle, Switzerland.

Introduction

Peter Joel Hurwitz

וכפטיש יפצץ סלע – מה פטיש זה מתחלק לכמה ניצוצות אף מקרא אחד
יוצא לכמה טעמים
בבלי סנהדרין ל"ד א

"And like a hammer that breaketh the rock in pieces" (Jeremiah 23:29): i.e., just as [the rock] is split into many splinters, so also may one biblical verse convey many teachings.

BT *Sanhedrin 34a*

WHY IS ASSISTED DEATH a topical worldwide problem nowadays?

The meteoric progress of medicine has gradually blurred the traditional boundaries between life and death, which up to a few decades ago were adequately characterized by the cessation of heartbeat and breathing. Today's mechanical and pharmacological support methods for circulation and respiration can maintain a person artificially and protractedly between life and death even when the brain, totally or in part, has failed irreversibly. A new definition of death has become unavoidable, and the concept of brain death has arisen, acquiring major significance also in transplant medicine. Today the criteria of brain death – the total and irreversible failure of all brain function – can be very precisely defined. Despite this, brain death is not universally recognized, and many religious and other groups continue to reject this definition of death. The demarcation lines between the proponents and opponents of brain death as a concept often cut across the various religions.

The possibility of delaying death for some time by medical means can be a mixed blessing. Sometimes, the term of life thus gained is so replete with unbearable suffering and pain that many patients no longer wish it and beg their doctors to cease treatment, accelerate death, or even kill them in order to curtail the suffering. We are thus faced with difficult questions that demand a balanced consideration of diverse value concepts. Is the technical maintenance of life at any price and in all circumstances justified, necessary, or desirable, and must physicians really do everything feasible to this end, or are humans so autonomous that they can decide by themselves how to end their lives, even when assisted suicide or requested killing are involved? How can we achieve a thoughtful equilibrium between these two extremes? How can we preserve human dignity, quality of life, and respect for the patient's wishes, so that prolonging life does not, under some circumstances, lead to nothing but prolonged agony, and so that the liberal use of pain-killers or the cessation of therapeutic procedures will not be interpreted as culpable manslaughter?

What is the duty of the physician? Is it to prolong the patient's life even against the latter's wishes, or to help in fulfilling the patient's wishes even if this means supplying death on demand? How do nurses assess these questions, given that they spend more time than the doctor with the patient and not infrequently see things in a different light? What is to be done when the patient, the patient's family, the doctors, and the nurses hold different views? What is to be done in the case of an incapacitated or unconscious patient, or of children and newborns? Can a person, while well and of sound mind, dictate a will that is legally binding in the event of incapacity at life's end? Who should advise a terminal patient on these questions, and how is the advice to be tendered? To what extent should the family be involved? And above all, how can abuse be prevented? These issues have ethical, religious and philosophical, social, medical, legal, and also – at a time of ever more limited means – economic aspects that raise ethical questions and require a comprehensive legal framework. All of society shares this problem, and it is no longer acceptable to leave the decisions, without clear guidelines, solely to the doctors. New legislation, acceptable to all or at least most of society concerning terminal care and assisted death, is now being discussed in many countries, and some have already enacted comprehensive new laws.

Why the Jewish Viewpoint?

The Jewish religion is not concerned solely with regulating relationships between man and God and between man and man; Jewish law also determines the behavior of the individual in all the activities of daily life. In Judaism, all that we now call constitution, statutes, civil law, and criminal law is embodied in the religious legal code, or Halakhah. Jewish law is based both on the Hebrew Bible, above all the Five Books of Moses (Torah in its narrower sense), and on the Talmud, a compilation of discussions and commentaries on the Mishnah, the body of postbiblical Jewish legislation. The material in the Mishnah was first handed down orally, then written down and codified in the second century C.E. The Talmud was codified and closed between the fourth and sixth centuries. The Five Books of Moses, the Mishnah, and the Talmud together are likewise called Torah in the wider sense (Torah meaning "teaching"). Legal interpretation and commentary have continued from the closing of the Talmud down to the present day by means of detailed rabbinic commentaries, written legal opinions, and adaptations to new situations. In order to render the entire process of origin, development, and adaptation of Jewish law more comprehensible, Rabbi David Bollag has written an introductory contribution on Jewish religious law.

The saving of human life has a very high priority in Judaism. "He who preserves one soul is considered as if he had preserved the whole world" (BT Baba Bathra 11a). In order to save one life one may, indeed one must, transgress all the commandments of the Torah except the three cardinal prohibitions of murder (literally: shedding blood, Hebrew: *shefihut damim*), idol worship, and sexual immorality. On the other hand, we are also commanded to prevent or to alleviate severe suffering . One may not hasten the onset of death, yet one may not delay it when it is imminent. This immediately offers some room for action, since the boundary between hastening death and not delaying imminent death is fluid. These fundamental considerations – preservation of life, avoidance of pain, and not delaying imminent death – can sometimes lead to a conflict of interests. For example, a mortally sick person who is suffering severely and pleads for treatment to be discontinued or indeed for death. Is life so sacred that everything humanly possible must be done to preserve it even for a few moments, in the face of untold agony and suffering, or, rather, are we fully autonomous with regard to the right to decide when our life should end? For both extreme positions and for all the intermediate shades of opinion there are advocates and opponents in Judaism.

Naturally these questions also engage non-Jewish society. However, for more than two thousand years Judaism has made legal decisions for all situations in life. These must constantly be interpreted anew for new and unprecedented circumstances, generally by drawing conclusions from analogies with comparable known situations. The basic laws are constant, but their interpretations can vary considerably. There is in Judaism no ultimate authority to rule on the correctness of a legal interpretation. Instead, respected rabbis, either on their own initiative or in response to third parties, make decisions on specific topics; these are then published in the form of *pesikot* (halakhic legal opinions) or as responsa (replies to queries). According to the Mishnah (Avot 1:6), Jews are commanded to seek out and attach themselves to a rabbi (a teacher, literally "one who has much knowledge"); one should go to the teacher in whom one has most confidence, but should not change him whenever there is disagreement with one of his decisions. Thus the rabbis and indeed all Jews have considerable freedom of decision and personal responsibility within the basic legal framework.

This book gives expression to the centuries-old tradition of debate and continuous legal reinterpretation and to the considered and diverse Jewish standpoints on the questions of life, suffering, and death. At the same time it adduces medico-ethical, philosophical, legal, and social reflections that constitute a contribution to the general and universal debate on this theme. The diversity of Jewish opinions and interpretations is reflected by the authors of this book, hailing from Switzerland, the United States, and Israel, and most of them acknowledged authorities in their fields. *The* Jewish opinion does not exist; rather, there are many and diverse views and interpretations.

This book is intended not only for special audiences – Jewish, medical, ethical, legal, or otherwise – but for interested general readers. Many of the concepts involved in this area are of universal importance irrespective of one's origin, religion, or outlook. The terms "active assistance" and "passive assistance," without precise definition and with a fluid transition between them, are today used with declining frequency. For example, is the omission of a treatment something passive, or is it not, in reality, an active decision not to prolong the patient's life?

Such concepts as the sanctity (inviolability) of life, quality of life, human dignity, autonomy, suicide, assisted suicide and termination of life on demand all require discussion and definition. This may lead to conflicts between civil law, religious, and ideological perceptions. In our age of great migrations, resulting in multicultural and multireligious societies which comprise many different minorities, this is particularly important and must be resolved with the widest possible social consensus. The right to make a medical will should be recognized, and writing such a document should be standardized and simplified. This would alleviate procedures with regard to terminal patients who are no longer of sound judgment. A good model for this, with the establishment of a central databank of advance medical directives, is presented by Avraham Steinberg in his essay on proposed legislation in Israel.

Palliative medicine is currently gaining in importance. Use of the right palliative means often achieves good pain therapy, thus avoiding the question of assisted death. Unfortunately, the role of palliative medicine in medical training and everyday practice is still far too small. Indeed, palliative medicine should be promoted more actively in the curricula of medical students, doctors, and care-givers, as well as in adjacent areas such as philosophy, law, and pastoral care.

We have avoided as far as possible using the term "euthanasia," principally because of its misuse during the Nazi era. The word "euthanasia" stems from ancient Greek and means "a good death," death in a good and agreeable manner, that is, in good spirits, without pain and suffering. This concept appears also in the Talmud in a discussion about execution of the death sentence. The term used there is *mitah yafah*, which means "a good death," that is, a condemned person is to be granted a good death. Rashi, living in France in the eleventh century and one of the most famous Bible commentators, answers the question as to what this would be with the words "that he might die quickly" (*sheyamut maher*), that is to say, that the condemned suffer as little as possible. In modern French legal parlance about assisted death, the term used is also *bonne mort* (see below, the contribution by Hofstetter and Marti).

Although the term "assisted death" is better than "euthanasia," it is equally inadequate. After all, the point is not merely to alleviate suffering for a desperate patient wracked by pain and at life's end, nor is it to facilitate or hasten the onset of death. Rather, the dying patient must be *given care*, indeed must *be accompanied*, for whether we influence the process of dying or not, the final period before death should be rendered as easy and agreeable as possible. Besides medical treatment and pain relief, this means, above all, personal contact with the dying, taking time to converse, to listen attentively, and as far as possible also to attend to the next-of-kin. In our general hospitals, where everyone is short of time, how often have we seen a dying patient for whom nothing more can be done, lying in bed, lonely and isolated? The daily doctors' round tarries briefly at the patient's bedside, and the participants are relieved to hurry on to "more urgent" matters. When I was a young resident in a rural hospital, I was most impressed by our farming people as patients. On their deathbed, they mostly wanted to go home and spend their last days among family. Just as we see our household guests to the door, so must we accompany the dying to their exit with dignity and love.

Structure of the Book

Rabbi David Bollag is an Orthodox rabbi, born in Basle and now living in Jerusalem. He provides a summary of the origins, development, and application of Jewish religious law from its biblical beginnings to the present day.

Dr. Elias Hofstetter and Mario Marti from Bern present a comparative study of the legal situation with regard to assisted death in various European countries and the United States.

Rabbi David L. Bleich of Yeshiva University, New York, is an international authority on Jewish law and ethics and has written numerous articles and books on bioethics and Jewish law. He represents a strictly Orthodox viewpoint.

Rabbi Leonard Kravitz of the Hebrew Union College in New York has published several studies on Jewish bioethics and is a representative of Liberal Judaism.

Rabbis Bleich and Kravitz both base the exposition of their viewpoints on biblical and talmudic sources as well as the extensive responsa literature. These sources do not speak explicitly of assisted death as it is understood today. However, they do contain a number of accounts and episodes which suggest some parallels to assisted death, and by the typical argument from analogy already mentioned, these can be applied to modern situations. But the same sources often lead the two rabbis to quite different interpretations and conclusions.

Professor Avraham Steinberg is a doctor and medical-ethicist in Jerusalem. He was the chairman of a government commission in Israel tasked with elaborating a draft law on the care of terminal patients. He reports on the origins of the commission, its composition, procedures, and deliberations, and includes dissenting minority opinions. The text of the draft law is presented beginning on page 215.

Dr. Vardit Ravitsky of the Department of Philosophy at Bar-Ilan University, Ramat Gan, describes some situations of conflict between the democratic basic legislation of the Jewish state and Jewish religious law.

Professor Shimon Glick, a physician, is a medical ethicist at Ben-Gurion University. As an Orthodox Jew he tries to find an acceptable synthesis of the often divergent opinions on the care of the end-of-life patient.

Rabbi Maurice Lamm, of Yeshiva University, New York, and founder and president of the National Institute for Jewish Hospice, emphasizes the importance of feeling and empathy when dealing with the dying.

Lydia Goldschmidt is a qualified nurse and head of nursing care at the Shaarei Zedek Medical Center, Jerusalem. She also teaches medical ethics and legal aspects of medicine at the Henrietta Szold School of Nursing at the Hebrew University Medical School, Hadassah Hospital, Jerusalem. Her contribution recounts her personal experiences as a nurse in a large municipal hospital in Jerusalem, where Jewish, Muslim, and Christian Arab patients are treated along with many war wounded and Jewish and Arab victims of terror.

For the sake of completeness, two non-Jewish authors have been invited to contribute.

Professor Hans Küng is a former lecturer on ecumenical theology at the University of Tübingen and founder of the Weltethos Foundation. He discusses the subject of assisted death in depth and presents his conclusions.

Professor Walter H. Hitzig is a hemato-oncologist and former head of department at the University Children's Hospital in Zürich. He writes about the terminal care of child cancer patients and cites, among other matters, a number of impressive instances of art therapy with mortally sick children.

This book deals with the complex problems of assisted death from many different angles. It is our intention to show that Judaism, despite being so strongly determined by laws, still allows for many different and sometimes even opposing viewpoints.

I wish to express my thanks to Prof. Jacques Picard for his valuable advice.

I dedicate this book to my wife, Nina, whose suggestions and advice contributed much to get this project started.

Jewish Religious Law

Rabbi David Bollag

H ALAKHAH, the term now used to denote the body of Jewish religious law, is a Hebrew word meaning "to walk." It expresses the aim of Jewish law, which is to accompany the Jewish person on his way through life, implying that he live his life according to its prescriptions.

One of the most characteristic features of Halakhah is to attend at every step in a Jew's life, even the apparently most profane. Jewish religious law comprises regulations, in the literal sense of the word, from cradle to grave, from the first to the final moments of life, from birth until death. "From before birth until after death" would be a more appropriate expression, because contraception, abortion, gene technology, and stem-cell research, as well as post-mortem examination and organ donation, are all problematic areas confronted by the Halakhah and subject to its decisions.

Thus Jewish religious law includes much more than so-called ritual matters. Of course these too constitute an integral, fundamental, and essential component of Judaism. Prayer, the Sabbath, the festivals, as well as kashrut, the laws governing food, are all indispensable components of Jewish religious practice. Halakhah is not, however, restricted to these areas, and, in its concern for all sides and aspects of human life, it also necessarily addresses and decides on the issues of assisted death and terminal care.

Jewish religious law is founded on Divine revelation. Halakhah is primarily a body of law given by God – in philosophical terms, it is heteronomous. This distinguishes it from, and to an extent contrasts it with, autonomous law, which is man-made and based on human reason alone. Nevertheless, many Jewish philosophers of religion throughout the ages have taken pains to emphasize that there is never a contradiction between Halakhah and human reason, which is to say that it is never irrational. On the contrary, Halakhah may be understood and explained rationally and is in complete consonance with human reason.

For example, the prohibition of murder in the Decalogue does not differ from the prohibition of murder found in human ethical systems. The origins of the prohibitions differ, but their content is the same.

According to Orthodox Jewish tradition, the commandments of the Torah, on which today's Halakhah is based, were revealed by God to the Jewish people at Mount Sinai more than three thousand years ago. Now it is clear that the commandments were revealed with reference to that era. Questions of Halakhah that arose in the ensuing centuries out of new circumstances, developments, and discoveries receive no explicit mention in the Sinaitic Law. Nevertheless, the commandments revealed then and anchored in the Torah have formed the basis of Jewish religious law to the present day, for they provide the principles and criteria by which new questions are resolved. The fields of technology and medicine, above all, have made huge progress in the last hundred years, and this progress has led to a plethora of halakhic questions.

The basis for the solution of novel halakhic problems is the principle of analogy. Contemporary halakhic authorities will endeavor to compare new, as yet unresolved problems to existing halakhic rulings, in order to adopt the considerations and decisions they apply and to use them in solving the new problem. This was the approach to questions arising out of the advent of electricity, and it is the approach to the attempted resolution of halakhic problems in modern medicine.

The complexity of many halakhic questions arises from the multiplicity of factors and aspects which must be considered in the process of argument and decision-making. Thus it is understandable that divergent halakhic decisions may often result, and that two rabbis may arrive at contrary conclusions for the same query. Both are correct and acceptable in that their authors both regard the commandments of the Divine revelation at Mount Sinai as the essential basis and the obligatory starting point for the treatment of halakhic questions.

The very complexity of many halakhic questions, particularly in the field of medicine, often causes a rabbi's *pesak halakhah* (religious-legal decision) to be very individual in nature. As the product of halakhic deliberations, it must take into account a multiplicity of criteria and factors about the specific situation. With questions of a medical nature, the considerations that enter the process of decision-making must include psychological, economic, sociological, and sometimes sociopolitical factors in addition to the medical facets.

Thus, abstract discussions of halakhic ordinances are often of only theoretical significance, because they treat and answer specific questions without reference to the environment. They are *in vitro* decisions. Of course they have a role to play *in vivo*, but in the process they often undergo significant restriction, expansion, and alteration.

The aim of this chapter is to present an overview of the content and history of Jewish religious law. The most important halakhic works and their authors will be introduced and briefly described. The presentation is arranged chronologically but should not be regarded as a history of the Halakhah. Instead, our primary purpose is to present and clarify the religious and theological basis, the sources, external influences, and inner mechanisms, involved in modern halakhic decision-making.

TORAH

The Five Books of Moses, the Pentateuch, form the basis of all halakhic ordinances. Jewish religious law recognizes 613 positive and negative biblical commandments. All 613 are to be found in the Pentateuch.

The other sections of the Jewish Bible, or Old Testament, are of little halakhic importance relative to the Pentateuch. These other sections, the books of the Prophets and the Writings (the Hagiographa), do occasionally play some role in halakhic discourse, but it is both qualitatively and quantitatively very limited. None of the biblical commandments originates from the Prophets or Writings, and no essential aspect of any commandment stems from these parts of the Bible. Only the Pentateuch is of primary importance for the birth and development of the Halakhah.

The Five Books of Moses are often called the Torah and are frequently referred to as the Five Books of the Torah. The word *torah* means "instruction" and expresses the Torah's purpose of guiding us on our way through life.

The term Torah is not always used only in this narrow sense. Sometimes the whole Bible is denoted as Torah. In a halakhic context, however, the name Torah is frequently used in a much broader sense, denoting the literature of Halakhah as a whole. All the works composed over the ages in the field of Halakhah are known *in toto* as Torah.

The Pentateuch serves as the foundation for the structure of all these works. Nevertheless the Five Books of Moses contain only a small fraction of the information required for the comprehension and application of the biblical commandments. For example, the prohibition of work on the Sabbath that is mentioned in the Decalogue is incomplete, because it does not define what is meant by work. Does the prohibition mean to forbid those activities on Shabbat by which we normally earn our living? Does it intend the interdiction of all strenuous physical actions – or perhaps something else?

In the view of Orthodox Judaism, God revealed the 613 commandments at Mount Sinai and instructed Moses exactly how to record them in writing. At the same time, for each commandment, God gave Moses explanations necessary for its application and comprehension. Thus He informed Moses, among other things, that the prohibition of labor on Shabbat comprises thirty-nine different acts of work, namely those performed during the construction of the Tent of Meeting in the desert, and analogous acts.

The part of the ordinances recorded in the Five Books of Moses is known as the Written Torah or Written Law. The additional explanations are called the Oral Law or Oral Tradition because they were not intended to be written down and were originally passed on by word of mouth down the generations.

The rise of Liberal Judaism began some two hundred years ago, and for the sake of simplicity, we will include the contemporary Reform and Conservative movements in that term. Their conception of the origin and development of the Torah is fundamentally different and represents the view that a considerable part of the Written and Oral Torah does not go back to a Divine revelation but is of human authorship, and above all, that what Orthodoxy calls the Oral Law arose only much later, after the destruction of the Second Temple.

Orthodox Judaism, however, adheres to the tenet that the Oral Tradition originated at Mount Sinai and explains that this part of the Sinaitic Tradition was not to be committed to writing in order to ensure a transmission free of errors. Information handed down orally can always be checked for having been correctly understood, with the possibility of corrective intervention. Thus, in Orthodox thought, the Torah falls into two mutually dependent and complementary parts: the Written Torah, being the Five Books of Moses, and the Oral Torah, which will be presented in detail below.

MISHNAH

For some fifteen hundred years the Oral Law was handed down from generation to generation without being recorded in writing. Individual scholars presumably made private notes as a memory aid, but these were intended only for personal use and were not published.

The compass of the Oral Tradition greatly increased during this time. After forty years of wandering in the desert, the Jewish people entered their land, where they created their own state, established a kingdom, and built a Temple. They faced many novel situations, for some of which exact instruction was available in the Sinaitic Law. However, for a significant part of these unprecedented situations new decisions had to be made. These new halakhic decisions on the most varied religious, political, and economic questions were all absorbed into the Oral Tradition, and their compass has grown steadily.

With the destruction of the Second Temple in 70 C.E., a new, very perilous situation arose for the Jewish population of the Land of Israel. The Temple, which had been the religious and spiritual center uniting them, no longer existed, and the Romans, a major political and military power, ruled the land with an iron hand. Among other things, they forbade the Jews under pain of death to study Torah and thus endangered the complete and sound transmission of the Oral Tradition.

Although Jews in considerable numbers ignored the prohibition of Torah study, tradition weakened so considerably with time that the loss of important parts of the Oral Tradition was widely feared. Rabbi Yehudah Hanasi (R. Judah the Prince), head of the Jewish community in Palestine at the end of the second century C.E., therefore decided, after thorough deliberation, to commit it to writing. He was fully aware that this was a breach of the original prohibition against writing down the Oral Law, but in view of the emergency, he justified the infringement as right and essential in order to ensure the intact transmission of the Torah.

Rabbi Judah the Prince had an extraordinary memory. He knew the whole Oral Law by heart, with a complete overview of its contents. He knew which scholar had handed down or innovated which decisions and where disagreements existed between the authorities; relying on his memory, he committed the Oral Law to writing.

Rabbi Judah's work is called the Mishnah. The word means "study" and "repetition," and refers to the prime function of the Mishnah text as the vehicle for study and rehearsal of the Oral Torah.

From what we have said, it is clear that Rabbi Judah the Prince did not so much write the Mishnah as write it down. He was not the author but the editor of the Mishnah. His labor, and his tremendous achievement, lie in his having collected the entire contents of the Oral Torah and prepared it for publication. He eliminated repetitions and whatever material he regarded as superfluous, and gave the final material a thematic arrangement.

The Mishnah is made up of six mains sections, known in Hebrew as *sedarim* ("orders"). These are divided into tractates (*massekhtot*), and these again into chapters. The Mishnah comprises a total of sixty-three tractates.

All the material that was part of the Oral Law at the time of Rabbi Judah the Prince but, for one of the reasons mentioned, was not included by him in the Mishnah is known as *baraita*, an Aramaic word meaning "outside, external." We will have more to say about the baraita below.

The prescriptions of Jewish religious law appear in the Mishnah as "case law." This means that halakhic rulings are presented for quite specific cases without explanation of the fundamental rules or principles behind them. What is more, the Mishnah is very laconic and is indeed formulated in key-word style. Rabbi Judah decided on this style of recording the Mishnah because his prime purpose was simply to save the Oral Law from oblivion. The Mishnah is an extremely brief memory aid to the Oral Law and always required a parallel commentary for its full comprehension.

TALMUD

The Mishnah achieved its purpose within a very short time, and was accepted everywhere as a reliable and authoritative collection of the Oral Law. In Palestine and also in Babylon, where large and important Jewish centers had existed since the destruction of the First Temple, the information in the Mishnah now became the starting point for religious-legal discussion and for consideration of every halakhic question.

Now, as we have said, this information was formulated not in full but rather as key-words. Because any written statement can be variously interpreted and understood, a lively debate about the correct interpretation of the Mishnah arose soon after its publication. All the prominent rabbis at the great academies in Palestine and Babylon participated in the discussions, presenting their opinions and arguments. These debates, conducted orally, were not recorded; they acquired the status of Oral Law and were handed down as such.

However, just as with the Mishnah itself, the concern gradually prevailed that these discussions, which had grown in importance and volume, might be forgotten, and again the decision was taken to record Oral Law. In Palestine the discussions in the academies were committed to writing toward the end of the fourth century, and in Babylon, at the turn of the fifth century and the beginning of the sixth. This written record of the interpretation of the Mishnah is known as the Talmud ("learning" in Hebrew). The Talmud composed in Palestine is known as the Jerusalem Talmud (JT), and that in Babylon, as the Babylonian Talmud (BT).

The Talmud was not carefully edited in the modern sense and should be regarded as a loose collection of discussions. As a result, it often contains repetitions, overlapping material, and also, frequently, contradictions. By whom and when the Talmud was composed is not entirely clear. In the current scientific view it was assembled by various scholars over a number years or even decades.

Although a talmudic discussion always starts from the Mishnah, the Talmud differs fundamentally from that work. While the Mishnah, in key-word style, wishes merely to save the most essential data of the Oral Law from oblivion, the Talmud aims at the most comprehensive analysis possible of the whole Oral Tradition, drawing all relevant aspects of the Mishnah into the discussion. The Talmud seeks to discover the reasons behind the rulings of the Mishnah, to understand the abstract and theoretical principles underlying the mishnaic case law. In contrast to the Mishnah, it also seeks to examine the connection between the Written and the Oral Torah, to ascertain what biblical commandment lies at the base of each mishnaic ruling, and to uncover the integral connection between the Written and the Oral Law.

To achieve all these ends the Talmud often has resort to the baraita, Oral Law material that existed at the time of the Mishnah but was not included therein by R. Judah the Prince. Indeed the Talmud endeavors to collect all the materials that are relevant, even in the widest sense, to the study, comprehension, and transmission of the total Torah. Thus the Talmud is often regarded as an encyclopedia of the Oral Law and forms to this day the basis of all halakhic discussion.

In the Talmud we find all the religious rulings of that time and all the arguments and decisions relevant to them. Orthodox Judaism regards these arguments and decisions as fully valid and binding to the present day.

The Talmud also differs linguistically from the Mishnah. The latter is in Hebrew, whereas the former is largely in Aramaic and partly in Hebrew. The Jerusalem and Babylonian Talmudim are both incomplete in the sense that no Talmud has come down to us for many tractates of the Mishnah and, indeed, for large parts of some orders. To this day it has not been established definitively whether the missing tractates had no Talmud or whether this material has been lost.

A very large and important part of the Talmud, known as the aggadah, is devoted to the discussion of questions not of direct relevance for Halakhah. As this essay concerns the history of Jewish religious law, we will devote no further discussion to this nonhalakhic part of the Talmud.

Within a short period, the Babylonian Talmud achieved overwhelming importance in comparison to the Jerusalem Talmud. There were three reasons for this. In the first place, the Babylonian Talmud had to a degree undergone better redaction and thus is easier to study. Second, the Babylonian Talmud was composed somewhat later and thus has greater halakhic authority, for in disputes between two scholars of the same epoch, the Halakhah decides according to the later opinion. The reason given is that the later scholar was aware of the earlier one's opinion and presumably had good grounds for disagreeing with it, whereas the earlier scholar might have adopted the later opinion had he known it. The third reason for the preeminence of the Babylonian Talmud is that during the ensuing centuries, the large Jewish centers in Babylon achieved incomparably greater importance than those in Palestine. The religious and spiritual center of Jewry had moved to Babylon, with the result that the Babylonian Talmud played a far more significant role in the further development of the Halakhah than did its Jerusalem counterpart.

Many centuries later, long after the invention of printing, the pagination system of the so-called Vilna Shas, an edition of the Babylonian Talmud printed in Vilna, prevailed. In consequence, source references to the Babylonian Talmud conventionally use these page numbers.

CODIFICATION

Like the Mishnah, the Talmud acquired almost unlimited authority soon after its publication. Traditions, arguments, and above all decisions recorded in the Talmud were, on principle, not to be contradicted. Halakhic rulings included in the Talmud were regarded as authoritative.

However, for a very large number of halakhic questions, the Talmud provides no decisions. Many questions are analyzed and thoroughly debated without reaching a decision. The Talmud is not very convenient as a source of information on halakhic decisions, and the need arose for the compilation of halakhic codes. The primary purpose of these works was to gather all questions of religious law and bring them to a decision.

There was a further reason for the need to codify. Although the Mishnah has a thematic structure which is thus imposed on the Talmud, the latter's contents display very little system. Talmudic discussion is frequently very associative in nature, allowing digression to lead from one topic to another. Thus, many topics are addressed in more than one place in the Talmud, which makes the integrative consideration of those questions extremely difficult. This too led to the need for codification of talmudic law – that is, for it to be collected, arranged in thematic order, and presented systematically.

In the course of about a thousand years after the conclusion of the Talmud, a number of codes were compiled – during the first five hundred years in Babylon, and in the later period, in North Africa and Europe. Very roughly speaking, the Babylonian codes have played only a minor role in the further development of the Halakhah, whereas the codes written in the second five hundred years are of major significance. The four most important of these will now be introduced.

Alfasi

Rabbi Yitzhak of Fez (Morocco, 1013–1103), known as Alfasi (Arabic for "of Fez"), was the first scholar of his time to try to decide all the halakhic questions raised in the Talmud. For this purpose he compiled a text parallel to the Talmud into which he inserted those passages of the Talmud that were, in his opinion, of halakhic relevance, and this text was to serve as a code. Parts of the Talmud discussing nonhalakhic questions were not included in his work. Where the Talmud decides a question, he adopts its decision and usually reproduces it verbatim. Where the Talmud cites various opinions on a question, he decides it by citing only the view he favors and omitting mention of the conflicting opinions. Likewise, he usually omits from his text the arguments brought by the Talmud, and he very rarely justifies his decision.

It should be noted that Alfasi does not address the many ordinances no longer practiced since the destruction of the Temple and the expulsion of the Jews from Palestine. Furthermore, he represents the Sephardic halakhic tradition – the tradition of the Jews of the Orient, North Africa, and Spain, a tradition which stems from Babylonian Jewry.

Maimonides

The legal code of Moses Maimonides (1135–1205), also known as Rambam, the great philosopher and halakhist who lived in Spain, North Africa, Palestine, and Egypt, differs fundamentally and in many ways from Alfasi's. The only feature they have in common is that Maimonides too absorbed and codifies the Sephardic tradition.

The greatest difference lies in the arrangement of the halakhic rulings. Maimonides, a totally systematic thinker, classified and arranged them in a completely new manner. He assembled, as it were mentally, the entire contents of the Talmud and all other relevant halakhic sources, classified them afresh, weighed them up, and made and recorded his decisions. His code, which he called *Mishneh Torah*, and which is also known as the *Yad Hazakah* ("Strong Hand"), is divided into fourteen books. Each of these is devoted strictly to one subject; the third book, for example, to the Sabbath and festivals. Each book is divided into subtopics; thus, one part of the third book covers Shabbat, and other parts are devoted to each of the festivals. Each of these parts is subdivided into chapters according to strict criteria. Maimonides' code is thus the first in which all the rulings on a subject are lucidly assembled and presented.

Two other noteworthy features distinguish this work from Alfasi's. First, Maimonides included both the halakhic rulings concerning the Temple service and the rulings that apply only when the majority of the Jewish people lives in the Land of Israel, wishing to compose a code that would be valid for all times. Furthermore, he intentionally devoted the first of his fourteen books to philosophical topics. For Maimonides, at least a little philosophy constitutes an integral part of Halakhah.

Although it was undisputedly a magnificent achievement, Maimonides' code was very strongly attacked and criticized. He was reproached even for his choice of the title *Mishneh Torah*, or "Second Torah," because it implies that his code is second in importance to the Torah and thus undermines the importance of the Talmud. His manner of codification was also roundly attacked. He was accused of adopting only his own opinions for his code, without citing his talmudic or other sources and without naming the scholars whose opinions he accepted. Despite all this censure, the monumental significance, authority, and quality of Maimonides' code has never been questioned.

Rosh
Rabbenu Asher (Rosh, 1250–1327) is the only purely Ashkenazic codifier of his time; in other words, the only one representing the tradition of North European Jewry, which lived mainly in Germany and northern France. He was himself one of the tosafists, a group of important commentators on the Talmud, and his halakhic decisions reflect the tradition and thinking of that school.

In his method, Rosh is close to Alfasi. Thus he deals only with halakhic problems relevant to the post-Destruction period and in the order of their appearance in the Talmud. He frequently gives his decision without extensive explanation, although he justifies himself more often than does Alfasi.

Rosh lived in Germany at a time of frequent and often very brutal anti-Jewish persecutions. Seeing no future for Jewry in Germany under these conditions, he sent his sons to study Torah in the talmudic academies of Spain. We will now turn our attention to one of these sons.

ARBA'AH TURIM

The third son of Rosh was Ya'akov ben Asher (ca. 1270–1340). In his father's house in Germany he grew up in the Ashkenazic tradition with regard to both religious practice and the intellectual approach to Torah study. His arrival in Spain as a young man brought him in contact with the Sephardic tradition, by which he was strongly influenced. His code includes both Ashkenazic and Sephardic traditions, with the influence of the latter emerging particularly in his method.

Sephardic Torah scholarship had always been distinguished by its more systematic character. For his codification of Jewish religious law, Ya'akov ben Asher felt compelled, like Maimonides, to abandon the fairly random organization of the talmudic material and to arrange the whole corpus of Halakhah afresh. He organized his work into four divisions, with the title *Arba'a Turim*, an allusion to the four rows (called *arba'ah turim* in the Torah) of precious stones on the breastplate of the High Priest. Like Maimonides, he devoted each division ("row") to a specific area, but his systemization is not as thorough. Each row is subdivided into paragraphs (*simanim*).

This work is usually referred to briefly as the *Tur*. Like Alfasi and Rosh, it codifies only halakhic rulings currently applicable. As seen from today, the importance of the *Tur* lies less in its quality or originality than in the influential role it played in the ensuing history of Halakhah codification.

SHULHAN ARUKH

Among the Jews expelled from Spain in 1492 was a four-year-old boy called Joseph Caro. Like so many others among the exiles, he journeyed through many lands of the Mediterranean basin, together with his parents and later by himself, finally settling in Tzefat (Safed) in northern Palestine.

The prevalent mood of the Jewish people in the years following the expulsion from Spain was one of disaster, reminiscent of the mood in the period following the destruction of the Second Temple, a mood which had ultimately spurred the compilation of the Mishnah. The great center on the Iberian Peninsula, where Jewry had flourished for centuries, had been destroyed, and all seemed doomed to destruction. On the religious front there was widespread concern about the apparently renewed danger to the transmission of the Torah. Jews were fleeing, often in small groups, to settle in diverse countries, and the maintenance of contact with other parts of the Jewish people was threatened. This could easily result in the isolation of many Jewish communities: uniform transmission and practice of the Torah would become impossible, and survival of the Jewish tradition would again be threatened.

The youthful scholar Rabbi Joseph Caro experienced and recognized this peril, which he resolved to counter. He made it his goal to compose a halakhic work that would unite all segments of the Jewish people and thus ensure the survival of the Torah.

His own opus he molded in the form of the *Arba'a Turim* and as a commentary to it with the title *Bet Yosef* ("House of Joseph"), a name intended to express the method and purpose of the work. Like the biblical Joseph, who had gathered all the corn of Egypt for survival during the famine years, he, another Joseph, would collect all the available halakhic material in his work and thereby promote the survival of the Jewish people in the era of the expulsion .

In the *Bet Yosef*, Caro assembles all the halakhic material relevant to every ruling in the *Tur* from the Pentateuch, through the Mishnah and Talmud, to the great codes. He analyzes and discusses the rulings and opinions, and in every case comes to a decision. However, this does not rest on his own deliberations but on the majority principle. Caro regards Alfasi, Maimonides, and Rosh as the greatest and weightiest halakhic authorities and therefore adopts the view of the majority among these three codifiers.

Concluding his work after more than thirty years, Caro realized that it would actually not achieve his goal. His commentary on every ruling in the *Tur* was so extensive, and required so much careful study, that only scholars would have the time and stamina to consult it. He therefore decided to write a supplementary work in which he would record only his halakhic decisions, to be called *Shulhan Arukh*, literally "A Table Laid." Metaphorically, the name suggests that the Halakhah is presented like food ready for consumption, in a manner directly applicable and not requiring further study. To facilitate use of the work, Caro adopted the *Tur's* four divisions and its subdivision into paragraphs. Anyone studying a specific item in the *Tur* or the *Bet Yosef* will thus find the ruling on it at the same location in the *Shulhan Arukh*.

In a very short time the *Shulhan Arukh* succeeded in becoming the accepted, authoritative, and binding code. Its sole drawback was that it usually presented the Sephardic tradition and ignored the Ashkenazic. A younger contemporary of Caro living in Cracow, Rabbi Moshe Isserles (1525–1572), undertook to write a supplementary commentary to every paragraph of the *Shulhan Arukh* where the Ashkenazic traditions differ from the Sephardic ones, indicating the difference and supplying the Ashkenazic ruling. These supplementary glosses contributed substantially to the rapid acceptance of the *Shulhan Arukh* as the universally binding code of the Halakhah which it has remained to this day.

The *Bet Yosef* likewise contributed to this success because anyone wishing to follow the complete process of decision leading to a halakhah in the *Shulhan Arukh* can do so by consulting the *Bet Yosef* on that item. This could not be done using Maimonides' *Mishneh Torah*, for example.

The mood of doom that prevailed in the period following the expulsion from Spain also played a part in this success, for the *Shulhan Arukh* filled the need which the mood had engendered.

Another decisive factor, in our opinion of no minor import, was the invention of printing. The *Shulhan Arukh* appeared at a time when, thanks to printing, a book could easily be put on the market in large numbers and widely distributed.

All these factors lie at the root of the undisputed authority of the

Shulhan Arukh to this day, so much so that any discussion of Jewish religious-legal questions must still pay prime attention to the opinion in that work. In the solution of new halakhic problems, the *Shulhan Arukh* plays a large and often, indeed, a decisive role.

RESPONSA LITERATURE

As a halakhic code, the *Shulhan Arukh* is binding to this day, but life and its halakhic implications have not stood still since the sixteenth century. Huge political and sociological changes have occurred that directly affect Jewish life. The intervening scientific and medical discoveries and the technical progress associated with them have continuously raised novel and complex halakhic problems.

Since the publication of the *Shulhan Arukh*, with its almost unassailed authority, the responsa literature has largely been the vehicle of new halakhic decisions. Under this system, specific halakhic problems arising from new situations are presented to recognized rabbinic authorities with a request for a written reply, a form known as a responsum.

Responsa are usually based on a comprehensive analysis of all the relevant halakhic material. The authority to whom the question is addressed is expected to master all the sources from the Torah, the Mishnah and Talmud, the codes, and the *Shulhan Arukh* that are required for a reply. In addition, he must have sufficient knowledge of the technical, medical, legal, and economic aspects to reply authoritatively on the question. We therefore frequently find specialization among the rabbis. One will deal mainly with medical questions, and another with electrotechnology. As we pointed out at the outset, newer halakhic responses are usually based on considerations of analogy with previously decided questions, and the replies are by no means always uniform.

The question of which rabbi's decision prevails is most complex and, however often asked, is difficult to answer. Jewry today has no supreme judicial body with the authority to make halakhic decisions that will obligate all Jews. Which rabbi's opinion is accepted depends on many and diverse factors. Of course the authoritativeness and clarity of argument and proof leading to the decision play a large role. Yet the rabbi's personality and his interpersonal abilities are also crucial, and sociological and political factors are often important. The process by which a responsum emerges as dominant is very dynamic, depends on many factors, and is not at all formalized.

JEWISH ETHICS

Finally, at this point we wish to raise the question of whether Halakhah and ethics are identical, or to what extent they coincide. It is clear and beyond dispute that Halakhah and ethics have much in common. Both Jewish religious law and general secular ethics have the greatest respect for human life Yet it is neither clear nor obvious that every ethical consideration must have immediate halakhic relevance and that every question of importance to Halakhah is always to be regarded as an ethical question. We therefore leave unanswered the question of whether Halakhah should be called "Jewish ethics." Jewish religious law is certainly ethical, but the identity of Halakhah and ethics still leaves room for profound deliberation.

References for Further Study

Albeck, Hanokh. *Einführung in die Mischna* (Berlin: de Gruyter, 1971). Trans. from the Hebrew ed. (Jerusalem, Mosad Bialik, 1959).

Elon, Menachem. *Jewish Law* (Philadelphia: Jewish Publication Society, 1994).

Encyclopaedia Judaica (Jerusalem: Keter, 1972), s.v. "Codification of Law," "Halakhah," "Mishnah," "*Shulhan Arukh*," "Talmud."

Feldman, David M. *Marital Relations, Birth Control, and Abortion in Jewish Law* (New York: Schocken, 1974), chap. 1.

Jüdisches Lexikon (Berlin: Jüdischer Verlag, 1927–30), s.v. "Halacha," "Halachot," "Schulchan Aruch," "Talmud."

Krupp, Michael: *Der Talmud* (Gütersloh: Gütersloher Verlagshaus, 1995).

Sammter, A. *Einleitung zu "Die sechs Ordnungen der Mischna"* (Basel: Goldschmidt, 1968), vol. 1, pp. xi–xiii.

Steinsalz, Adin. *The Essential Talmud* (New York: Basic Books, 1976).

Steinsalz, Adin. "Talmud." In *Contemporary Jewish Religious Thought*, ed. Arthur A. Cohen and Paul Mendes-Flohr (New York: Charles Scribner's Sons, 1987). <<provide author's name and put in proper alphabetical place in list>>

Stemberger, Günter. *Einleitung in Talmud und Midrasch* (Munich: Beck, 1992).

Assisted Death

A STUDY IN COMPARATIVE LAW

Elias Hofstetter and Mario Marti

I. INTRODUCTION

1. Topics and Objectives

The aim of the present contribution is to introduce the reader to the current legal limits of assisted death and assisted suicide and to their "limited flexibility."[1] This will create the basis for an informed and detailed discussion of the subject, and such discussion necessitates rudimentary acquaintance with the legal situation – at least in a state founded on the rule of law.

For this purpose and bearing in mind the international nature of the readership, we will consider some different legal systems. A fairly detailed description of the legal situation in Switzerland is followed by a survey of that in Holland, France, and the United States. The resulting observations will enable us to draw some conclusions, including several of a comparative legal nature.

2. Terminology: Assisted Death and Assisted Suicide

It is obvious that the legal systems considered here do not all use exactly the same classifications. However, the following definitions, intended as an aid for orientation on the subject, have been chosen with sufficient breadth to include solutions other than the Swiss as freely as possible. The fundamental distinction between assisted death and assisted suicide is important for an understanding of this essay.

Assisted death can apply in principle only to the *dying,* "persons who, to the satisfaction of a physician on the strength of clinical indications, suffer from a disease or traumatic injury that is irreversible and will, despite treatment, lead to death in a foreseeable time."[2] However, the term *assisted death* is also used where there is "severe cerebral damage with irreversible, focal or diffuse brain injuries resulting in a chronic vegetative state."[3]

The concept of assisted death is further divided into *actively* and *passively* assisted death, with the further distinction that actively assisted death can be brought on *directly* or *indirectly. Direct(ly) actively* assisted death implies "a treatment" (usually by medication) in the sense of deliberately killing the suffering patient.[4] In contrast, *indirect(ly)* actively assisted death involves the curtailment of the patient's (remaining) life as a possible secondary and calculated consequence of an objectively necessary treatment (e.g., the administration of pain killers, "aggressive palliative treatment"), the purpose of which is to alleviate suffering. On the other hand, authors and legal decisions in certain countries, such as the United States,[5] adopt a subjective approach and require the purpose of pain relief to be the decisive element.

Direct actively assisted death, already mentioned above, is also sometimes linked to an intention, namely "an intention to kill." In the typical case, this intention itself is fundamentally a "final" decisive diminution of suffering, which indeed involves terminating a life of affliction. In the extreme case and final resort, the difference between an immediately lethal injection, given for the sole purpose of relieving pain (and for no other reason), and a pain-killing medication with a probable life-curtailing effect of greater or lesser intensity, is only a graduated difference between a greater and lesser abbreviation of the time left to live, that is, between a faster and slower onset of death.[6]

The term *passively assisted death* is used when life-prolonging or -maintaining measures are waived in the case of a patient who is dying or in a state of prolonged vegetation. Except for some possibly palliative measures, no further treatment is undertaken or any such existing treatment is discontinued (e.g., by switching off a heart-lung machine).[7] A case of assisted suicide can only arise when a person wishing to die, whether well or sick, brings about his death *himself*, (the so-called power to act or the autonomy of action of the suicide).[8]

II. LEGAL SITUATION IN SWITZERLAND

1. Current Law

1.1 LEGAL EMBODIMENT

Legal formulation of assisted death must start from fundamental legal principles. The rights to life, personal freedom and the protection of human dignity are constitutional rights.[9] From these fundamental principles derives the right to self-determination of every patient, and with it, every person's sole prerogative to decide himself about fate of his own body.[10]

The outcome of these principles in criminal law is the fundamental prohibition of killing the other, the basis and sanction of which are found in the criminal law code.[11] The norms established in this codification concern in a general way the criminal law's appraisal of a case of death under extraneous influence. However, neither in this code nor in other legal sources valid today do we find actual regulations formulated specifically for assisted death.

1.2 CRIMINAL LAW FORMULATION

In appraising assisted death, authoritative criminal law distinguishes between several types of cases (cf. above, 1.2):

a. Direct actively assisted death

Actively assisted death means the deliberate killing of a dying person. Such an action, as the injection of a patient with a lethal substance, satisfies the factual requirements for deliberate homicide according to Art. 111 StGB.[12] The agent's noble motives or the hopeless situation of the patient can alter nothing with regard to the punishable nature of the act, nor, basically, can the wishes of the patient do so (see, however, 1.2.d below).[13] No superordinate grounds exist for justifying the act of assisting death. Thus an action carried out in the sense of actively assisting death leads necessarily to the punishment of the person assisting the death. Consideration of the motives will, if at all, follow during sentencing.

b. Indirect actively assisted death

Administering pain-relieving drugs to a critically ill patient may, as a side-effect, facilitate or accelerate the onset of death. If a doctor administers such a drug knowing its possibly lethal side-effect, he is accepting the demise of the patient. The fatal result, only indirectly wanted, and despite this its acceptance, is known in theoretical criminal law as possible intent. This is treated in the same way as direct intent with regard to the facts of the case. An act performed out of possible intent is thus liable to the punishment for that act with intent. Thus, also in the case of indirect assisted death we find affirmation of the circumstance of homicide. Nevertheless, in practice and with the assent of theory, punishment has been waived for such offenses. Protecting a patient from unbearable pain is regarded as a common-law professional duty of the physician.[14] This allows a defense plea according to Art. 32 StGB, i.e., the act is justified because its performance is required by professional duty.[15]

However, narrow limits have been imposed on the permissibility of using such medications. It has been recognized only when the medication is *essential* for the relief of pain.[16] This criterion would be satisfied only when the patient is suffering the severest pain and no other analgesic with less risky side-effects can be given.[17]

c. Passively assisted death

In contrast to actively assisted death, demise of a person under passively assisted death is the result not of action but of omission. This brings to mind particularly the failure to carry out a life-prolonging treatment, e.g., by withholding a critical medication.

Besides the result of the act and its performance, criminal liability for an offense of dereliction requires that the offender was legally obliged to carry out the act that he omitted. Thus, the offender must have been duty bound to prevent the resulting occurrence to the best of his ability.[18] This so-called *status of trustee* toward the person willing to die may be deduced from the legal duty to give succor and, particularly, from published legislation on emergency aid by doctors.[19] The treating physician acquires the status of trustee toward the patient merely on the grounds of the Agreement to Treat concluded with the patient.[20] This gives rise to the principle that killing a person by failing to act is culpable homicide. We should note, however, that there is some tension between the doctor's status of trustee and *the right to self-determination* of the patient. The right to self-determination gives the patient exclusive power to make decisions about his body. This right includes the possibility of forgoing a treatment which is medically indicated and essential for life. A decision such as this, which can lead ultimately to the death of the patient, is to be respected by the medical team. The doctors then have no right to treat; indeed, the patient also has a right to medically unsound treatment. If the doctor is obliged to respect the wishes of the patient and to refrain from what is actually essential treatment, no criminal blame can attach to the doctor in the event of the patient's death. The patient has, to a degree, withdrawn himself from the protection of the doctor, who is therefore relieved of any obligation of action or trusteeship.

In this connection there is an important restriction: in order for his waiver of treatment to be valid, the patient must be *competent to judge.*[21] If a person is capable of reasonable action, he is also competent to judge and can decide freely about his treatment. It is, however, essential as a preliminary that the patient be fully informed by the treating physician about the consequences and risks of his decision. With the true situation of the patient and his needs being taken into account, the patient is to be put into a situation which allows him to make his decision on the basis of free and exhaustive information.[22]

If a person lacks the competence to decide, his actions cannot, in principle, have any legal consequences,[23] nor can a life-maintaining procedure then be legally dispensed with. The utterances of a person incompetent to decide are therefore not binding on the doctor. Instead of the person *incompetent to decide*, his legal representative (parent, guardian) decides in the first instance. Life-sustaining measures may be neither interrupted nor denied against the will of these representatives.[24] On the other hand, the decision by the legal representative to waive life-sustaining measures is only binding when it is oriented to the welfare of the child[25] or the ward. If the legal representative rejects the undertaking of medical procedures, his opinion is to be overruled by the medical team if it is an abuse and obviously not in the interest of the rationally incompetent patient.[26]

The question arises in certain cases whether a person incompetent of judgment and without a legal representative should be treated. In that situation, a decision to conduct or omit treatment can be made neither by the person concerned nor by a legal representative, so that the decision to treat or desist from treatment devolves on the doctor. For this decision the professional must rely on the *presumed wishes of the patient*.[27] The presumed wishes of the patient should be ascertained on the basis of all the circumstances of the patient's life and can be determined from conversations with the patient's family and friends. Advance medical directives (AMD), in which patients as yet competent to judge make advance decisions for the time when incompetence to judge may supersede, are not absolutely binding on the doctors, but they do represent a strong presumption as to the estimated will of the patient,[28] and they will be ignored only in those exceptional cases where there is overwhelming evidence for a change of mind by the patient.

d. Death on demand

The principle of punishment for killing another person is not basically altered even when the patient explicitly demands death at the hands of the doctor or terminal caregiver. Admittedly, the circumstances (according to Art. 111 StGB) of premeditated killing then no longer apply and give way to the mitigating circumstances of killing on demand, according to Art. 114 StGB. Such mitigation does not absolve from penalty but affects only its degree. The difference originates in the demand made by the person wishing to die and, in order for the mitigation of Art. 114 StGB to apply, this demand must be "serious and forceful," Mitigation of the penalty is furthermore conditional on the presence of "worthy motives" on the part of the offender. The law cites pity as an example of a worthy motive. If such motives cannot be proven, and instead, self-seeking motives are found to play a decisive role, the mitigation lapses.

It can thus be maintained that in current law, neither the wishes of the patient nor elevated motives for the killing affect the fundamental criminality of assisted death.

e. Assisted suicide

It is a consequence of the patient's right to self-determination that in penal law, a suicide attempt is not punishable. It follows from this that aid to that offense, normally punished less severely, is not penalized in this case. There is one exception to this principle in Art. 115 StGB: assistance to suicide is explicitly punishable if there is a presumption of attendant self-seeking motives. The helper to a suicide is thus only punishable if he extends this help in order to attain a personal advantage.

Whether the behavior of the doctor or a third-person party to the death of the patient is to be judged as premeditated killing or as assistance to suicide is itself a criminal-law decision depending crucially on the question whether the person wishing to die had or did not have freedom of action with regard to his own death.[29] If he has the power to perform the killing, e.g., he takes the lethal medication himself, then he commits suicide. However, if the final act is ascribed to the helper, suicide is absent, and the rules of actively and passively assisted death must be applied.

1.3 PROFESSIONAL APPRAISAL

In 1995 the Swiss Academy for Medical Sciences promulgated medical-ethical guidelines for the medical care of the dying patient and of patients with extreme cerebral damage ("SAMW-Richtlinien, [guide lines]" revised 2003), as well as medical-ethical guidelines for the care of terminal patients (revised 2004). These guidelines define the conditions under which passively assisted and indirect actively assisted death are permissible.[30] Actively assisted death is prohibited explicitly.[31] To render aid to suicide is denoted as "being no part of medical activity,"[32]

The guidelines of the Swiss Academy for Medical Sciences are an integral part of the Professional Rules of the Union of Swiss Physicians. Basically these are *not* a matter of State law but rather of private law (Association Rules). Thus, infringement of professional rules does not entail state sanctions, and professional measures can be imposed instead. By contrast, a criminal judge will judge the assisted suicide solely on the basis of the relevant criminal-law rulings. The professional rules may serve as aids in the interpretation of the state law.[33] The medical-ethical guidelines for the medical care of the dying patient and of patients with extreme cerebral damage are sometimes indirectly granted the quality of norms. Thus, in Canton Bern, the Regulations on Assisted Death and Determination of Death[34] declare the Guidelines to be applicable.

2. Current Debate

On the political level Switzerland has seen several initiatives aimed at bringing about a change in the law.

In 1994, National Councillor Ruffy demanded a relaxation of the present penal rulings. A moderated version of the initiative was sent to the Federal Council in 1996, and it appointed a working group that later elaborated proposals for (new) legislation ("Report of the Working Group on Assisted Death").

The working group is unanimously of the opinion that passive and indirectly active assisted death should be regulated by law, but has refrained from formulating a proposal. The following is its fundamental position:

PASSIVELY ASSISTED DEATH:

Anyone abstaining, at the request of a patient, from taking life-pro-longing measures is not (continues not to be) punishable, irrespective of the patient's condition or medical prognosis.

INDIRECT ACTIVELY ASSISTED DEATH

In the opinion of the working group, there is valid justification for this on the grounds of professional duty (Art. 32 StBB) not only when the doctor recognizes life-curtailment as a possible side-effect, but also when this seems to him to be as good as certain.

As to the admissibility of actively assisted death, opinion in the working group is divided. A small majority holds that Art. 114 StGB should be complemented in §2 by a new clause which will exempt the offender from punishment in the case of *extreme exceptions.* These are to be found when the patient's health is incurably impaired and as-sisted death represents the only means for releasing the patient from unbearable pain and irremediable suffering.

The Federal Council, in giving its opinion on the Report of the Working Group, favored the promotion of palliative medicine and an explicit regulation of passively and of indirect actively assisted death (Federal Council's Report on Assisted Death). The Federal Council however, refused on grounds of principle to relax the prohibition of homicide in granting exceptional admissibility of direct actively as-sisted death, a step which it called a breach of taboo.

After several other parliamentary initiatives were proposed and some were approved by Parliament,[35] the debate around assisted death and suicide has continued.

III. FOREIGN LEGISLATION

At this point we will briefly survey a few legal systems and thus pro-vide a broader perspective for the formulation of further possible solutions.

A. CONTINENTAL EUROPE (CIVIL LAW)

1. The Netherlands

Dutch legislation on assisted death – first the Burial Law of 1994,[36] and later the supplementary Law on Assisted Death and Suicide of 2002[37] as well as the relevant decisions by the courts – is regarded in political debate as "progressive," insofar as it also permits actively assisted death under certain circumstances.

1.1 PASSIVELY ASSISTED DEATH

In recognition of the patient's right to self-determination, passively assisted death, as currently defined, is apparently permitted. Authority lies with the wishes of the patient. If the patient can no longer express himself, "sole responsibility for an action for or against cessation of treatment or abandonment of further rescue procedures, devolves on the doctor treating the case. Thus, the near-of-kin have no say whatsoever. This represents a considerable deviation from legislation in the neighboring countries."[38]

1.2 INDIRECTLY ASSISTED DEATH

Treatment, life-shortening but necessary as a palliative, is permissible. This was recognized by Dutch jurisdiction long before the legislation on assisted death came into force.[39]

1.3 DIRECT ACTIVELY ASSISTED DEATH

Actively assisted death remains basically punishable both under the Burial Act of 1994 and the Law on Assisted Death and Suicide of 2002 (Art. 293 Paragraph 1 NL StGB).[40] It is exempt from penalty only if carried out on the express wish of the patient and additionally under certain factual and procedural conditions. The conditions necessary for impunity have remained basically the same since 1994. The new 2002 Law on Assisted Death and Suicide has the following to say about them (Art. 2):

1. In order to comply with the due-care criteria referred to in article 293, paragraph 2, of the Criminal Code, the attending physician must:
a. be satisfied that the patient has made a voluntary and carefully considered request;
b. be satisfied that the patient's suffering was unbearable, and that there was no prospect of improvement;
c. have informed the patient about his situation and his prospects;
d. have come to the conclusion, together with the patient, that there is no reasonable alternative in the light of the patient's situation;
e. have consulted at least one other, independent physician, who must have seen the patient and given a written opinion on the due care criteria referred to in a. to d. above;
and
f. have terminated the patient's life or provided assistance with suicide with due medical care and attention.

2. If a patient aged sixteen or over who is no longer capable of expressing his will, but before reaching this state was deemed capable of making a reasonable appraisal of his own interests, has made a written declaration requesting that his life be terminated, the attending physician may comply with this request. The due care criteria referred to in subsection 1 shall apply *mutatis mutandis*.

The procedure is still regulated by the Burial and Cremation Act, which requires that the presence of the above conditions be recorded on a standard form. Between 1997 and 2002, five interdisciplinary committees, composed of doctors, lawyers, and ethicists, handed the State Attorney's Office a recommendation about the conformity of medical practice with the rules in the individual case.[41] The state attorney was thus to be notified of every case of assisted death. The Law of 2002 provided for the continued existence of the commissions. What is new is that no notification is made if the commission raises no objection to the doctor's procedure. Thus the work of the commission has actually gained in importance.

Originally the High Court based the above exemption from penalty on the presence of an emergency-like conflict of duties.[42] It was only in 2002 that the Law on Assisted Death and Suicide led to a specific modification of the penal code (Art. 293, Paragraph 2).[43]

1.4 ASSISTED SUICIDE

Assisted suicide is (still) fundamentally punishable (Art. 294 Paragraph 2 NL StGB[44]),[45] but criminal prosecution has been waived since 1994[46] in cases where conditions prevail in the same sense as those relevant to assisted death (see above, III.A.1.3) Again, the Act of 2002 finally brought about the corresponding adaptation of the penal code by excluding this act from criminality (Art 294 Paragraph 2 NL StGB). As to the presumptions for exemption from penalty, the said norm refers, *mutatis mutandis,* to Art. 293 Paragraph 2 NL StGB, which norm itself refers back to Art. 2 of the Assisted Death and Suicide Law (*due care*). It is thus clear that impunity is granted only in an assisted suicide which satisfies the strict demands of *due care* (incurable disease, suffering, etc.).

2. France

French criminal law (as yet) contains no specific regulations on assisted death. Several draft laws have been rejected, and some are pending.[47]

2.1 PASSIVELY ASSISTED DEATH

Passively assisted death is, in principle, not punishable because the regulations of the new criminal code (*nouveau code pénal,* NCP) penalize only murder and homicide committed by an action, i.e., as a deed,[48] and it is precisely this which is absent in passively assisted death. The situation thus resembles that of Swiss law, for example. But in contrast to the latter, French law does not recognize the non-genuine offense of commission by omission ("*commission par omission*").[49] A *prohibition,* the order to refrain from a certain deed, is therefore never interpreted by the French courts as a *command to act*, as a requirement to do a deed.[50] It is only the legislator who has the right, by means of explicit wording, to render an omission punishable, i.e., a real omission (*"pure omission"*). The legislator has used this authority in the enactment of the rule concerning the failure to render help (Art. 223–6 al. 2 NCP).[51] The applicability of this norm to the case under discussion is disputed. According to what is probably the prevailing opinion, a "moral" obligation to give succor (*"aider le mourant à mourir,"* "helping the dying to die [i.e., peacefully]) exists even when, in the absence of any possibility of rescue, death will soon follow.[52] Against this, others hold that the existence of at least a minimal chance for rescue is necessary, and therefore that no obligation to act exists in criminal law in the case of people who, even with rendered aid, will die inevitably and within a short time.[53]

2.2 INDIRECT ACTIVELY ASSISTED DEATH

When, in order to relieve pain, a doctor administers drugs which can curtail life (*"bonne mort,"* "a good death") to a suffering and dying person, the literature will justify this as an emergency. There are very few if any legal decisions on this question.[54]

2.3 DIRECT ACTIVELY ASSISTED DEATH

Direct actively assisted death, irrespective of the patient's will, is punishable as premeditated homicide (*meurtre*) or even as aggravated homicide (*assassinat*) (Art. 221–1, Art. 221–3 NCP):

> Le consentement de la victime est…indifférent dans la mesure où le meurtre est réprimé dans l'intérêt de l'ordre public avant d'être la conséquence du dommage causé à la victime. On retrouve donc ici…le cas du meurtre sur demande dans l'euthanasie…
>
> (The consent of the victim is…of no consequence insofar as homicide is curbed primarily in the public interest and only then because of damage done to the victim. Thus we again find…the case of murder on request in euthanasia …).[55]

There are no mitigating circumstances for killing on request as there are, for example, in Swiss law. The worthiness of the motive or the demand made by a patient is a matter for the judges to consider in regard to penal leniency (Art. 132–24 NCP).[56] In conformity with this, the *code de déontologie médicale* (Code of Medical Practice) likewise forbids a doctor intentionally to curtail the remaining life of the dying (Art. 38).[57]

2.4 ASSISTED SUICIDE

French criminal law punishes encouragement to suicide that "includes an active element and shows a link to 'incitement'"[58] (Art. 223–13 NCP).[59] There are as yet no further rulings in the *nouveau code pénal* about suicide or assistance to suicide, except for the prohibition to solicit the means to suicide, etc., a matter irrelevant to our subject. We may deduce from this that suicide itself and mere assistance with it are not punishable.

B. UNITED STATES (COMMON LAW)

1. Development of Legislation

In the United States, there has been scientific and public debate on questions of assisted death since the mid-seventies.[60] As responsibility for criminal and civil legislation lies primarily with the individual states of the federal United States, it is within their mandate to legislate about assisted death.[61] In those instances where they have legislated at all beyond the traditional bounds of homicide, the individual states have used this mandate in the most varied manners. An additional difficulty for the *civil law lawyer* is that in the matter of assisted death, *statutory law* and *case law*, itself a characteristic feature of *common law*, are heavily intertwined, and *case law* continues to wield the most influence.[62] However, on the whole, the U.S. law on assisted death and suicide can be deemed more restrictive than its continental European counterpart. Attempts to legalize suicide and actively assisted death in the United States seem to have met with no success so far except in the State of Oregon. However, here too there is an apparent tendency to "liberalize" the law on assisted death.[63]

2. Current Legal Situation

2.1 PASSIVELY ASSISTED DEATH (*VOLUNTARY EUTHANASIA*)

In the United States, a patient capable of rational decision is entitled to refuse a treatment or have it discontinued at any time.[64] Legal opinion has deduced this right from the constitutionally guaranteed protection of privacy and from the right to self-determination. However, a high level of proof is required to show that the right to self-determination is being satisfied and that genuine *informed consent* pertains:

> More acutely even than in our own legal environment, mere proof of consent…is insufficient. American case law demands a consent founded on clearly comprehensible information which is both detailed and refers specifically to the affected patient. Consequently, it is insufficient for the doctor to attend on and appraise the process of therapy or death, on his own professional authority: rather, he is obliged to supervise the individual stages of the sickness while maintaining, as it were, a continuous exchange of information with the patient.[65]

In exceptional cases, legally defined limits can be set to the right to self-determination when overwhelming public interests are involved, such as protection of life, protection of third parties, and the integrity of the medical profession, for example when a patient refusing treatment would have a good chance of recovery by means of surgery or therapy.[66]

Meanwhile each state of the Union has enacted laws mostly known as Natural Death Acts or Living Will Statutes, which regulate the admissibility and form of advance dispositions made by patients (advanced health-care directive) for the event of their future incapacity to judge.[67] These variegated legislations present a picture of confusing diversity.[68] Characteristically for Anglo-American legislation, most of them have in common a very detailed regulation of the form and legal wording of the directive that refuses life-supporting measures in the event of irreversible coma. In fact, the patient's wish to refuse life-supporting measures is not explicitly binding on the physician according to all state legislations except Oregon. The wording of the relevant regulations absolves him from a prison sentence only in the case that he obeys the wish of the patient.[69]

An institution remarkable in the view of Continental European jurists is that of the *attorney-in-fact*. This is a person in a position of trust who is authorized to make binding declarations of intent on behalf of the authorizing party in the event of the latter becoming incapable of such declaration (*durable power of attorney for health-care*). In Anglo-American law also, the power of attorney lapses when the authorizing party becomes incapable of action; several states have therefore legislated to continue the validity of such powers of attorney beyond the onset of incapacity to decide.[70]

If the patient is inarticulate and has prepared no *advance care health directive* or appointed no *attorney-in-fact*, the right to decision, according to one school of thought, devolves on another person (*surrogate decision-maker*). The latter must first of all acquaint himself with the presumed will of the inarticulate patient. Depending on the state, various persons (relatives, close acquaintances, doctors) are recognized as a *surrogate decision-maker*. In Massachusetts, it is the court that is authorized to decide. By means of this transfer of the power of decision to another person, this legislation wishes to convey that the patient has not been deprived of his basic rights, despite the loss of his ability to decide on these matters. The legislation by other states rejects this substitution and requires the existence of objective, legally predetermined criteria[71] for cessation of treatment.

Finally, it should be mentioned that the National Conference of Commissioners on Uniform State Laws (NCCUSL) has been trying since 1982 to halt the divergent legislation processes concerned with passively assisted death and with patients' dispositions, while recommending several alternative model laws for introduction by the states of the Union.[72] The NCCUSL's current legislative model is the Uniform Health-Care Decisions Act of 1993.[73]

2.2 INDIRECT ACTIVELY ASSISTED DEATH

Under certain circumstances, indirect actively assisted death is accepted as a secondary result of a medically indicated procedure. What matters here, as elsewhere, is the distinction between the intent to kill and an intent to palliate that merely takes the curtailment of life into account as an inevitable side-effect. Moreover, the appropriate palliative treatment must be required by the dignity of the person, who will otherwise suffer "undignified suffering."[74]

2.3 DIRECT ACTIVELY ASSISTED DEATH (MERCY KILLING)

Killing, even at the express demand of the patient, is judged to be murder (except Oregon which has a more lenient legislation). The nature of the patient's demand and the motives for the deed, e.g., pity (*mercy*), will at most be taken into account during sentencing.[75]

2.4 ASSISTED SUICIDE

Suicide is forbidden in most of the states of the Union, so that in these states assistance to suicide is likewise criminal, whether the motives be exalted or reprehensible.[76] The motive for rendering assistance will be considered only when the sentence is being decided. How consistently attempted suicide and assistance thereto are prosecuted by the authorities is a different question.[77]

IV. CONCLUSION

Assisted death is currently the subject of controversial political debate, at least in the industrialized countries of the international community of states. Appropriately, the problem is also in vogue in the relevant fields of medicine, law, philosophy, theology, and others. However, its very topicality complicates any comparison of the legal boundary conditions. On the national level, legal regulation of assisted death is in a state of flux; today's law is outmoded tomorrow. Legal systems that continue to prohibit actively assisted death are at present being subjected to a legislative activism which takes the form of close definition of the norms for assisted death (compare, for example, Sec. III B, United States). The question whether (direct actively) assisted death should *legally* be forbidden or allowed is not one which the legal disciplines (in the narrow sense) can or should be the first to answer. Primarily, the considerations underlying specific legislative decisions belong less to medicine than to philosophy, ethics, and theology. Jurisprudence and medicine will then have to work with the existing legal foundations. However, the courts will have "enhanced" importance as long as there are no specific regulations on assisted death. Thus many a legal debate about the latter will be decided by appeals to general teachings in its justification and, particularly, about "emergency" and other such issues.

From the point of view of jurisprudence, there is cause for reflection on at least one matter: Well-meant but hasty legislative activism often leads to ill-defined and contradictory regulations that are detrimental rather than favorable to legal certitude. The same is true for excessively detailed norms (lengthy enumerations and definitions), which of necessity elicit an interpretation equally "literal" or "clinging to the letter" and expose unsparingly the omissions of enumeration, that experience shows to be inevitable. In comparison, the existing law will often be preferable. Although it may be phrased in general terms and appeal, as we have shown, to general principles, the existing law usually has the advantage of proven use and worth. Naturally, those who desire a solution that differs from present practice, as, for instance, permission of actively assisted death where it has hitherto been forbidden, will espouse a different opinion.

We must treat with caution the division into "conservative," "liberal," or perhaps "progressive" assisted-death legislation (in the wider sense) that is the daily fare of politicians and the media. Holland, the paradigm of a country with "progressive" assisted-death legislation, does indeed permit actively assisted death under certain circumstances, but regards as criminal every form of assistance to suicide. Switzerland and France, on the other hand, prohibit actively assisted death but basically do not punish assisted suicide: the offender is only punished if he acts out of "self-seeking" motives (Switzerland) or incites to suicide, but not if he merely aids it (France). In the customary terminology, the Dutch law on actively assisted death proves to be more "liberal" than the Swiss, while the Swiss and French laws on assisted suicide are more "liberal" than the Dutch. Yet it would be both hasty and unjustified to conclude that these laws suffer from internal contradictions of judgment.

The subject of assisted death breaches the bounds of jurisprudence and medicine, For this reason, the examination of this topic *also* from a Jewish ethical perspective is much to be welcomed.

BIBLIOGRAPHY

Andreas Bucher, *Natürliche Personen und Perönlichkeitsschutz*, 3A (Basel: Helbing & Lichtenhahn, 1999).

Arbeitsgruppe Sterbehilfe, "Bericht an das Eidg. Justiz- und Polizeidepartement vom März 1999" (http://www.bj.admin.ch/themen/stgb-sterbehilfe/b-bericht-d.pdf) (quotes: Bericht Arbeitsgruppe Sterbehilfe).

Andreas Donatsch, "Die strafrechtlichen Grenzen der Sterbehilfe," *Recht* 2000, pp. 141 ff.

J.C.J. Dute, "Landesbericht Niederlande," in *Ärztliche Verantwortung im europäischen Rechtsvergleich*, ed. Gerfried Fischer and Hans Lilie (Cologne, Berlin, and Munich: Carl Heymanns Verlag, 1999), pp. 285 ff.

Hans Giger, *Reflexionen über Tod und Recht* (Zürich: Orell Füssli Verlag, 2000).

Karl-Ludwig Kunz, "Sterbehilfe: Der rechtliche Rahmen und seine begrenzte Dehnbarkeit," in *Festschrift für Stefan Trechsel zum 65. Geburtstag* (Zürich: Schulthess Polygraphischer Verlag, 2002), pp. 613 ff.

Mario Marti, "Sterbehilfe in der Schweiz," *Schweizerische Ärztezeitung* 83 (2002): 570 ff.

Anja Nussbaum, *The Right to Die: Die rechtliche Problematik der Sterbehilfe in den USA und ihre Bedeutung für die Reformdiskussion in Deutschland* (Strafrechtliche Abhandlungen, n. F. Bd. 128) (Berlin: Duncker & Humboldt, 2000).

Jean Pradel, *Droit pénal général*, vol. 9A (Paris: Editions Cujas, 1994).

Michèle-Laure Rassat, *Droit pénal spécial*, vol. 3A (Paris: Dalloz, 2001).

Jörg Rehberg, "Arzt und Strafrecht," in *Handbuch des Arztrechts*, ed. Heinrich Honsell (Zürich: Schulthess Polygraphischer Verlag, 1994).

Kathrin Reusser, *Patientenwille und Sterbebeistand*, Zürcher Studien zum Privatrecht, vol. 112 (Zürich: Schulthess Polygraphischer Verlag, 1994).

Antoine Roggo, *Aufklärung des Patienten: eine ärztliche Informationspflicht*, Abhandlungen zum schweiz. Recht: vol. 663 (Bern: Verlag Stämpfli & Cie, 2002).

David Rüetschi, "Ärztliches Standesrecht in der Schweiz – Die Bedeutung der Medizinisch-ethischen Richtlinien der schweizerischen Akademie der medizinischen Wissenschaften," in *Die Privatisierung des Privatrechts – rechtliche Ordnung ohne staatlichen Zwang*, Jahrbuch Junger Zivilrechtswissenschaftler 2002, ed. von Carl-Heinz Witt et al. (Stuttgart, 2003), pp. 231ff.

Hans-Joseph Scholten, "Landesbericht Niederlande," in *Materialien zur Sterbehilfe – eine internationale Dokumentation*, Beiträge und Materialien aus dem Max-Planck-Institut für ausländisches und internationales Strafrecht, Band s 25, ed. Albin Eser and Hans-Georg Koch (Freiburg im Breisgau, 1991), pp. 451ff.

Schweizerische Akademie der Medizinischen Wissenschaften, Medizinisch-ethische Richtlinien für die ärztliche Betreuung sterbender und zerebral schwerst geschädigter Patienten vom 27. November 2003, in *Schweizerische Ärztezeitung* 85 (2004): 50ff. (http://www.samw.ch/content/Richtlinien/d_RL_PVS.pdf) (cites: SAMW-Guidelines)

Schweizerische Akademie der Medizinischen Wissenschaften, Medizinisch-ethische Richtlinien zur Betreuung von Patientinnen und Patienten am Lebensende vom 25. November 2004, in *Schweizerische Ärztezeitung* 86 (2005): 171ff. (http://www.samw.ch/content/Richtlinien/d_RL_Sterbehilfe.pdf).

Schweizerischer Bundesrat, Bericht zum Postulat Ruffy, Sterbehilfe. Ergänzung des Strafgesetzbuches vom Juli 2000 (http://www. bj.admin.ch/themen/stgb-sterbehilfe/ber-ruffy-d.pdf) (cites: Bericht Bundesrat Sterbehilfe).

Margret Spaniol, "Landesbericht Frankreich," in *Materialien zur Sterbehilfe – eine internationale Dokumentation*, (eiträge und Materialien aus dem Max-Planck-Institut für ausländisches und internationales Strafrecht, vol. s 25, ed. Albin Eser and Hans-Georg Koch, Freiburg im Breisgau, 1991), pp. 281ff.

Günter Stratenwerth and Guido Jenny, *Schweizerisches Strafrecht, Besonderer Teil 1: Straftaten gegen Individualinteressen*, vol. 6A (Bern: Stämpfli Verlag, 2003).

Stefan Trechsel, *Schweizerisches Strafgesetzbuch vom 21. Dezember 1937: Kurzkommentar*, 2A (Zürich: Schulthess Polygraphischer Verlag, 1997).

G. van der Wal, "Evaluation of the Notification Procedure of Physician-Assisted Death in the Netherlands," *New England Journal of Medicine* 335 (1996): 1706ff.

Thomas Weigend and Alfred Künschner, "Landesbericht USA," in *Materialien zur Sterbehilfe – eine internationale Dokumentation*, Beiträge und Materialien aus dem Max-Planck-Institut für ausländisches und internationales Strafrecht, vol. s 25, ed. Albin Eser and Hans-Georg Koch (Freiburg im Breisgau, 1991), pp. 669ff.

Wolfgang Wiegand, "Die Aufklärungspflicht und die Folgen ihrer Verletzung," in *Handbuch des Arztrechts*, ed. Heinrich Honsell (Zürich: Schulthess Polygraphischer Verlag, 1994).

Jerry B. Wilson, *Death by Decision: The Medical, Moral and Legal Dilemmas of Euthanasia* (Philadelphia: Westminster Press, 1975).

Notes

1. Kunz, 613
2. SAMW-Guidelines (see Bibliography), Paragraph I, cf. also Paragraph II. 1.2
3. SAMW-Guidelines Paragraph I, cf. also Paragraph II. 1.2
4. Marti, 570

5. Vacco, Atty. General of New York, et al., v. Quill et al., 117 S.CT. 2293, 138 L.ED.2D (1997).
6. Thus also Kunz, 619: "The *inadequate delimitability* of the range in which indirect actively assisted death is applicable derives from the circumstance that the permitted risk of life-curtailment is arbitrarily high, reaching almost to certainty. Permissible reduction of suffering associated with a risk of life curtailment thus becomes practically indistinguishable from life curtailment which reduces suffering" (italics as in the original).
7. "Switching off" is, of course, an action; nevertheless, at least in Switzerland, the prevalent opinion is that the term "passively assisted death" includes it, for despite the element of switching off, abstention from or omission of further life-maintaining measures (a continuous medical intervention!) is the primary consideration.
8. Cf. below II.1.2.e
9. Cf Articles 7 and 10 of the Swiss Constitution (BV; SR 101) and Articles 2 and 5 of European Convention on Human Rights (ECHR).
10. The law of self-determination in its civil law formulation is to be found in Article 28 of the Swiss Civil Code (ZGB; SR. 210).
11. Article 111 et seq. of the Swiss Criminal Code (StGB; SR. 311.0).
12. Stratenwerth/Jenny, § 1 N. 8; Giger, 163; Donatsch, 143; Kunz, 618.
13. Rehberg, 317.
14. Ibid.
15. Giger, 164.
16. Rehberg, 317; Stratenwerth/Jenny, § 1 N. 8; Trechsel, N. 8 on Art. 111.
17. Kunz, 619.
18. Trechsel, N 32 on Art. 1.
19. Cf. e.g. Art. 30, Para. 1 of the Health Law of Canton Bern (BSG 811.01).
20. Rehberg, 318.
21. Art. 16 ZGB (Competence to judge): "Competent to judge is anyone who does not lack the ability to act reasonably on account of his minority or as a result of mental illness, mental deficiency, drunkenness, or similar circumstances."
22. On the question of elucidation, cf. e.g. Wiegand, 119ff., Roggo, 1ff., as well as the Professional Rules of the Union of Swiss Doctors (FMH) of 12 December 1996.
23. Art. 18 ZGB: "Legal exceptions aside, the actions of a person who is not competent to judge can have no legal consequences."
24. Cf. SAMW Guidelines Paragraph II./3.3
25. Cf. Art. 301 ZGB: "Parent conduct the care and education of a child with its welfare in mind and, with the reservation about the child's own competence to act, make the necessary decisions."
26. Bucher, 129, Rn. 528.
27. Rehberg, 319.
28. Reusser, 185.
29. Trechsel, N. 1 on Art. 115.
30. SAMW-Richtlinien Paragraph II. 1.2, 1.3, 2 and 3.
31. SAMW-Richtlinien Paragraph II. 1.4.
32. SAMW-Richtlinien Paragraph II. 2.2.
33. For the status of the Guidelines as legal norm, see, in detail, Rüetschi, 244ff.
34. BSG 811.06. The Guidelines are reproduced in the Appendix to the Regulation.

35. Parliamentary Initiative "Criminality of actively assisted death; legal revision" (00.441), submitted to the National Council by Franco Cavalli (Sept. 27, 2000; rejected by Parliament); Parliamentary Initiative "Encouragement of and assistance with suicide. Revision of Article 115 StGB" (01.407), submitted to the National Council by Dorle Vallender (Mar. 14,.2001; rejected by Parliament); Motion "Assisted death. To close the legal loophole rather than to permit killing" (01.3523), submitted to the National Council by Guido Zäch (Oct. 3, 2001); passed by Parliament). The last-mentioned charges the Federal Council with submission of a change in the law.
36. Burial and Cremation Act.
37. Termination of Life on Request and Assisted Suicide (Review Procedures) Act.
38. Giger, 233.
39. Verdict of the Leeuwarden District Court on Jan. 21,1973 ("Postma Case," NJ 1973, 183).
40. "Any person who terminates another person's life at that person's express and earnest request shall be liable to a term of imprisonment not exceeding twelve years or a fifth-category fine."
41. An appraisal of the reporting procedure is to be found in G. van der Wal, 1706 ff.
42. Cf. Dute, 285 as well as Scholten, 456 ff.
43. "2. The act referred to in the first paragraph [termination of life] shall not be an offense if it is committed by a physician who fulfills the due care criteria set out in section 2 of the Termination of Life on Request and Assisted Suicide (Review Procedures) Act, and if the physician notifies the municipal pathologist of this act in accordance with the provisions of section 7, subsection 2 of the Burial and Cremation Act."
44. "Any person who intentionally assists another to commit suicide or provides him with the means to do so shall, if suicide follows, be liable to a term of imprisonment not exceeding three years or a fourth-category fine. Article 293, paragraph 2, shall apply *mutatis mutandis.*"
45. It follows that inducement to suicide is all the more culpable (Art. 294 Paragraph 1 NL StGB).
46. Dute, 285 (referring to the then Burial and Cremation Act).
47. The draft bill (no. 3499) on the adoption of the right to die with dignity ('instituant le droit de mourir dans la dignité') of Dec. 19, 2001 as well as the draft bill (no. 788) on the right to end one's life in liberty ('relative au droit de finir sa vie dans la liberté') of Apr. 10, 2003 were returned to the preparatory commission. Both drafts permit actively assisted death under certain conditions. The draft of 2001 (Art. 1) requires, *inter alia*, that natural death would set in anyway within three months.
48. Art. 221–1 NCP: "Le fait de donner volontairement la mort à autrui constitue un meurtre…" (Ending the life of, or killing another person voluntarily or wilfully constitutes homicide.)
49. That is, according to the letter of the regulation, only a deed is forbidden (a prohibition). For a *genuine* offense of omission, on the other hand, the very formulation already penalizes a certain failure to act, passivity (an obligation to act).
50. Pradel, N. 364: "La règle de l'interprétation stricte interdit en effet toute assimilation d'une omission à une action positive seule prévue par la loi" (The rule of narrow interpretation [of criminal statutes] precludes the equation of a [passive] omission with a statutorily stipulated positive act). See also Rassat, N. 249.
51. "Sera puni des mêmes peines [cinq ans d'emprisonnement et de 75000 euros d'amende] quiconque s'abstient volontairement de porter à un personne en péril l'assistance que,

sans risque pour lui ou pour les tiers, il pouvait lui prêter soit par son action personnelle, soit en provoquant un secours" (The same punishment [five years of imprisonment and a fine up to 75,000 euros] is to be inflicted on anyone who knowingly refrains from assisting a person in danger when the assistance, posing no risk to the helper or third persons, could be provided by the helper personally or by his procuring rescue).

52. Rassat, N. 335, end.
53. Tribunal correctionel de Poitiers, Oct. 25, 1951, Juris-Classeur périodique 1952, vol. II, p. 6932 (still refers to the old regulation on rendering aid, Art. 63 Clause 2 CP). Cf. for all this also Spaniol, 287 f.
54. Spaniol, 295.
55. Rassat, N. 251
56. Spaniol (283) cites a report in Le Monde (Jan. 7, 1983, p. 12) according to which a man who out of pity had killed his suffering wife, sick with cancer, was sentenced to two years' prison on probation.
57. "Le médecin doit accompagner le mourant jusqu'à ses derniers moments, assurer par des soins et mesures appropriés la qualité d'une vie qui prend fin, sauvegarder la dignité du malade et réconforter son entourage.

Il n'a pas le droit de provoquer délibérément la mort" (The physician has to attend to the dying person until his last moments, and ensure by appropriate care and measures the quality of the life which is ending; he must protect the dignity of the dying and give comfort to those around him. He has no right wilfully to induce death).
58. Giger, 226.
59. "Le fait de provoquer au suicide d'autrui est puni de trois ans d'emprisonnement et de 45,000 euros d'amende lorsque la provocation a été suivie du suicide ou d'une tentative de suicide. "Les peines sont portées à cinq ans d'emprisonnement et à 75000 euros d'amende lorsque la victime de l'infraction définie à l'alinéa précédent est un mineur de quinze ans"

(Inducement of a person to commit suicide is punishable by three years' imprisonment and a fine of 45,000 EUR, if the inducement is followed by suicide or attempted suicide.

The punishment is up to five years of imprisonment and a fine of 75,000 euros if the victim of the above-mentioned offence is a minor of no more than fifteen years).
60. Weigend and Künschner, 671.
61. Nussbaum, 62 f.
62. Giger, 244.
63. Thus also Giger, 241, 243, 244.
64. See the opinion of the court (C.J. Rehnquist) in *Vacco, Attn. General of New York, et al. v. Quill et al.*, 117 S.CT. 2293, 138 L.ED.2D (1997); see also Nussbaum, 68 ff.
65. Giger, 245.
66. Giger, 248 f.
67. E.g., Washington's Natural Death Act (RCW 70.122).
68. See the Prefatory Note to the Uniform Health-Care Decisions Act 1993, as well Giger, 243.
69. Weigend and Künschner, 672.
70. Ibid., also on the difficulties associated with the conventional *durable power of attorney*.
71. See Giger, 251 ff. for the whole topic.

72. 1982: Model Health-Care Consent Act; 1985: Uniform Rights of the Terminally Ill Act; 1989: Uniform Rights of the Terminally Ill Act.
73. Online at http://www.nccusl.org; http://www.law.upenn.edu/bll/ulc/fnact99/1990s/uhcda93.htm.
74. Giger, 242; Weigend and Künschner, 671.
75. For a specific legal regulation, see, for example, Illinois Criminal Code of 1961 (720 ILCS 5), Sec. 9-1

    (First degree murder …): "(a) A person who kills an individual without lawful justification commits first degree murder if…(c) Consideration of factors in Aggravation and Mitigation. The court shall consider, or shall instruct the jury to consider any aggravating and any mitigating factors which are relevant to the imposition of the death penalty…Mitigating factors may include…the following:…(3) the murdered individual was a participant in the defendant's homicidal conduct or consented to the homicidal act…"
76. Cf. the elaboration by Chief Justice Rehnquist in *Dennis C. Vacco, Attorney General of New York, et al., v. Timothy E. Quill et al.*, 117 S.CT. 2293, 138 L.ED.2D (1997). See also, for example, New York Penal Law § 125.15 (Manslaughter in the second degree): "A person is guilty of manslaughter in the second degree when…(3) he intentionally causes or aids another person to commit suicide." Washington Criminal Code (RCW 9A.36.060) (Promoting a suicide attempt): "A person is guilty of promoting a suicide attempt when he knowingly causes or aids another person to attempt suicide."
77. Cf. on this: Wilson, 148 ff.

Treatment of the Terminally Ill

J. David Bleich

PRESERVATION OF LIFE

The Dilemma

Medicine has long subscribed to the adage "Thou shalt not kill; but needs't not strive officiously to keep alive."[1] Nevertheless, until relatively recent times, medical science was able to offer either all or nothing in its treatment of virtually all illnesses and diseases. Either the patient responded to treatment, when treatment was available, and was cured, or else he or she succumbed to the ravages of the malady. These dichotomous possibilities generated few moral dilemmas for the medical practitioner. Patients, by and large, sought treatment, and physicians strained to do all in their power to effect a cure. To be sure, theologians and ethicists agonized over such questions as the moral legitimacy of euthanasia for patients who found continued existence too painful to bear and the extent to which the patient was obliged to seek extraordinary means in effecting a cure; but the number of people with regard to whom such perplexities were germane was not nearly as great as in our day.

In recent years medical science and technology have made tremendous strides. Some diseases have been virtually eradicated; effective remedies have been found for others. Concomitantly, ways and means have been developed which enable physicians to sustain life even when known cures do not exist. As a result, issues concerning prolongation of the life of the terminally ill now arise with hereto-fore-unprecedented frequency. Economic considerations coupled with the stark reality of patients suffering from debilitating illnesses, and often incapable of engaging in meaningful or satisfying activities, have combined to create a milieu in which the focus of concern is upon quality of life.

The physician's practical dilemma can be stated in simple terms: to treat or not to treat. In deciding whether or not to initiate or to continue treatment, the physician is called upon to make not only medical but moral determinations. There are at least two distinguishable components that present themselves in all such quandaries. The first is a value judgment: Is it desirable that the patient be treated? Should value judgments be made with regard to the quality of life to be preserved? The second question pertains to the personal responsibilities of the physician and of the patient: Under what circumstances, and to what extent, is the physician morally obligated to persist in rendering aggressive professional care? Is the patient always obliged to seek treatment designed to prolong life even though a cure is not anticipated?

Jewish teaching with regard to these questions is shaped by the principle not only that human life in general is of infinite and inestimable value, but that every moment of life is of infinite value as well.[2] Accordingly, obligations with regard to treatment and cure are one and the same regardless of whether the patient's life is likely to be prolonged for a matter of years or merely for a few seconds. Thus, on the Sabbath, no less than on a weekday, efforts to free a victim buried under a collapsed building must be continued even if the victim is found in circumstances such that survival for longer than a brief time is impossible.[3]

Life with suffering is regarded, in many cases, as preferable to cessation of life and with it the elimination of suffering. The Gemara in Sotah 22a, followed by Rambam, Hilkhot Sotah 3:20, indicates that the woman required to drink "the bitter waters" (Numbers 6:11–31) did not always die immediately. If she was guilty of the offense with which she was charged but had some other merit, the waters did not cause her to perish immediately, but instead produced a debilitating and degenerative state which led to a protracted termination of life. The added longevity, although accompanied by pain and suffering, is deemed a privilege bestowed in recognition of meritorious actions. Life accompanied by pain is thus viewed as preferable to death. [4] This sentiment is reflected in the words of the psalmist, "The Lord has indeed chastened me, but He has not left me to die" (Psalms 118:18).

The practice of euthanasia, whether active or passive, is contrary to the teachings of Judaism. Any positive act designed to hasten the death of the patient is equated with murder in Jewish law, even if death is hastened by only a matter of moments. No matter how laudable the intentions of the person performing an act of mercy killing may be, the deed constitutes an act of homicide.

One nineteenth-century commentator finds this principle reflected in the verse "But your blood of your lives will I require; from the hand of every beast will I require it; and from the hand of man, from the hand of a person's brother, will I require the life of man" (Genesis 9:5). Fratricide is certainly no less heinous a crime than ordinary homicide. Why then, having already prohibited homicide, is it necessary for Scripture to prohibit fratricide as well? R. Jacob Zevi Mecklenburg, in his commentary on the Pentateuch, *Ha-Ketav ve-ha-Kabbalah*, astutely comments that, while murder is the antithesis of brotherly love, in some circumstances the taking of the life of one's fellow man may be perceived as an act of love par excellence. Euthanasia, designed to put an end to unbearable suffering, is born not of hatred or anger, but of concern and compassion. It is precisely the taking of life in circumstances in which it is manifestly obvious that the perpetrator is motivated by feelings of love and brotherly compassion that the Torah finds necessary to brand as murder pure and simple. Despite the noble intent that prompts such an action, mercy killing is proscribed as an unwarranted intervention in an area which must be governed by God alone. The life of man may be reclaimed only by the Author of life. So long as man is yet endowed with a spark of life, as defined by God's eternal law, man dare not presume to hasten death, no matter how hopeless or meaningless continued existence may appear to be in the eyes of a mortal.

Personal Autonomy
In stark contrast to the value system posited by Judaism, decisions in a series of cases handed down by American courts in recent years have upheld the right of a mentally competent adult to decline any and all forms of medical intervention even in instances in which it is clear that death will ensue. The sole recognized exceptions involve situations in which the adult is the parent of a minor child or in which intervention is necessary to preserve the life of a fetus. In such situations, earlier decisions have recognized the state's "compelling interest" in not allowing a situation to develop in which the child might become a ward of the state, and a number of decisions have recognized the state's interest in safeguarding the life and health of an unborn child.

The touchstone of a democratic society is the concept of individual freedom and personal autonomy. Democratic societies are quite properly dedicated to the maximization of personal freedom and find it necessary to justify any violation of personal privacy and any intrusion into the personal affairs of their citizens. These democratic traditions stand diametrically opposed to the absolutism which is the hallmark of the autocratic systems of government whose excesses cause so much human suffering.

No one will dispute the claim that personal freedom and individual autonomy are religious values. Yet it is readily apparent that, in a hierarchical ranking of values, the values of personal freedom and autonomy do not occupy a position within a religiously oriented ethical system identical to that which they occupy in a secular system of values. This certainly is the case insofar as Jewish tradition is concerned and serves to explain why a patient dare not refuse treatment clearly required to preserve life.

Judaism teaches that man has no proprietary interest either in his life or in his body. Our bodies and lives are not ours to give away. The proprietor of all human life is none other than God Himself. As Radvaz, Hilkhot Sanhedrin 18:6, so eloquently phrases it: "Man's life is not his property, but the property of the Holy One, blessed be He."[5]

According to Jewish teaching, the personal privilege and personal responsibility extended to the human body and to human life are similar to the privilege and responsibility of a bailee with regard to a bailment with which he has been entrusted. It is the duty of a bailee who has accepted an object of value for safekeeping to safeguard the bailment and to return it to its rightful owner upon demand. With regard to the human body, man is but a steward charged with preservation of this most precious of bailments and must abide by the limitations placed upon his rights of use and enjoyment. Thus any claim to absolute autonomy is specious.

This moral stance is reflected in the mores of society at large, although not to the same degree. Despite contemporary society's commitment to individual liberty as an ideal, it recognizes that this liberty is not entirely sacrosanct. Although there are those who wish it to be so, self-determination is not universally recognized as the paramount human value. There is a long judicial history of recognition of the state's "compelling" interest in the preservation of the life of each and every one of its citizens, an interest which carries with it the right to curb personal freedom. What the jurist calls a "compelling state interest" the theologian terms "sanctity of life." It is precisely this concept of the sanctity of life which, as a transcendental value, supersedes considerations of personal freedom. This is implicitly recognized even in the provisions of the Natural Death Act enacted in various jurisdictions; otherwise such legislation would grant citizens unequivocal authority to terminate life by any means and in all circumstances. Were autonomy recognized as the paramount value, society would not shrink from sanctioning suicide, mercy killing, or even consensual homicide, under any or all conditions.

Jewish tradition certainly recognizes liberty as a value but defines freedom and liberty in a very particular way. The mishnaic dictum *ve-lo atah ben horin le-hibatel mi-menah* (Ethics of the Fathers 2:16) is rendered by the fifteenth-century commentator R. Isaac Abarbanel, not in the usual manner as "nor are you free to desist from it" (i.e., from obedience to the law), but as "nor in desisting from it are you a free man." Freedom is the absence of constraint which would interfere with realization of man's potential. The laws of the Torah are designed to facilitate man's endeavors in fulfilling the Divine plan inherent in creation. Casting off the yoke of law is not an act of freedom but its antithesis. This concept is very similar to what the British philosopher T.H. Green called "positive freedom."

Liberty, as the term is conventionally understood, is a paramount value only when it does not conflict with other divinely established values. In secular terms, personal autonomy must give way to preservation of the social fabric. The state has an interest, which is entirely secular in nature, in the preservation of the life of each of its citizens. In the absence of other competing interests, it may assert its authority to compel the preservation of a life against the wishes of a citizen in spite of the deprivation of liberty entailed thereby because public policy accepts the moral thesis that the preservation of life must be regarded as a superior value, taking precedence over the right to privacy and the value of personal autonomy.

Yet as reflected in Jewish law, Judaism bestows a privileged position upon preservation of human life as a moral value in a manner unparalleled in other value systems. As a moral desideratum, it takes precedence over virtually every other value. Exceptions to the general rule that preservation of life takes precedence over all other considerations are transgression of the three cardinal sins for purposes of preserving life. These are murder (hardly an exception), idolatry, and sexual offenses such as incest and adultery. All other laws are suspended for purposes of conservation of life. Even the mere possibility of preserving life mandates suspension of biblical restrictions, however remote may be the likelihood of success in saving human life.

TREATMENT OF THE TERMINALLY ILL

Modes of Treatment: Natural vs. Artificial; Ordinary vs. Extraordinary

The foregoing discussion reflects the unique position that preservation of life occupies in the hierarchy of values posited by Judaism. Judaism regards human life as of infinite and inestimable value. The quality of the life that is preserved is thus never a factor to be taken into consideration. Nor is the length of the patient's life expectancy a controlling factor.

Since Judaism regards every moment of life as sacred, the patient is obliged to seek treatment, and religious laws are suspended for the sake of such treatment even if there is no medical guarantee of a cure.[6] Similarly, the physician's duty does not end when it is no longer possible to restore the lost health of the patient. The obligation "and you shall restore it to him" (Deuteronomy 22:2) refers, in its medical context, not simply to the restoration of health, but to the restoration of even a single moment of life. Again, Sabbath restrictions and other laws are suspended even when it is known with certainty that human medicine offers no hope of a cure or restoration to health. Ritual obligations and restrictions are suspended so long as there is the possibility that life may be prolonged even for a matter of moments.

Nevertheless, there remains considerable doubt in the Jewish community, and perhaps even a measure of disagreement, with regard to the permissibility of withholding various forms of medical treatment from the terminally ill. In Israel the matter has been exacerbated by the adoption of a statute exonerating physicians and any other persons from criminal liability "for a medical action or treatment performed with lawful permission of an individual for the person's benefit." In an attempt to dispel confusion, the following statement was issued recently by a group of leading Israeli rabbinic decisors:

According to the law of the Torah it is obligatory to treat even a patient who, according to the opinion of the physicians, is a terminal, moribund patient with all medications and usual medical procedures as needed. Heaven forfend that the demise of a terminal patient be hastened by withholding nutrients or medical treatments in order to lessen his suffering. *A fortiori*, it is forbidden to hasten his demise by means of an overt act (other than if it is clear that these are his last hours, in which case even movement [of the patient] is forbidden since he is a *goses*.)

Below is a list of medical treatments compiled by senior physicians.

In accordance with what has been stated above, it is incumbent upon the families of terminally ill patients to concern themselves

and to request that the patients receive treatment in accordance
with the above-stated principles.
 (Signed)
 Joseph Shalom Eliashiv   Shlomo Zalman Auerbach
 Shmu'el ha-Levi Woszner   S.Y. Nissim Karelitz

Appended to this statement is a list of mandatory treatments that includes intravenous or gastric feeding, IV fluid replacement, insulin
injections, controlled dosages of morphine, antibiotics, and blood
transfusions.[7]

Jewish law with regard to care of the dying is spelled out with
care and precision. The terminal patient, even when he is a *goes* – that
is, who has become moribund and whose death is imminent – is regarded as a living person in every respect. One must not pry his jaw,
anoint him, wash him, plug his orifices, remove the pillow from un-
derneath him, or place him on the ground.[8] It is also forbidden to
close his eyes, "for whoever closes the eyes with the onset of death is a
shedder of blood."[9] Each of these acts is forbidden because the slightest movement of the patient may hasten death. As the Talmud puts
it, "The matter may be compared to a flickering flame; as soon as one
touches it, the light is extinguished."[10] Accordingly, any movement or
manipulation of the dying person is forbidden. Furthermore, passive
euthanasia involving the omission of a therapeutic procedure or the
withholding of medication which could sustain life is also prohibited
by Jewish law. The terminal nature of an illness in no way mitigates
the physician's responsibilities, because the physician is charged with
prolonging life no less than with effecting a cure.

Although, as will be noted presently, there may well be some limitations upon the obligation to preserve life, many commonly asserted
moral distinctions have no basis in Jewish teaching. Any distinction
between "natural" and "artificial" means of treatment is without prec-
edent in Jewish law. Indeed, upon examination, the distinction is fundamentally specious. Medical substances synthesized in the laboratory
are certainly not natural, yet it is unlikely that ethicists would regard
such medications as artificial. For that matter, even drugs extracted

from plants and the like are hardly natural sources of nutrition for man but assuredly would not be classified as artificial. The obligation to revive a person from drowning is one of the paradigms of *pikuah nefesh* ("concern for human life") advanced by the Gemara, Sanhedrin 73a. That obligation includes the duty to throw a life preserver to the potential victim. In what sense is a respirator designed to deliver oxygen to the lungs different from the casting of a life preserver? A drowning person too exhausted to grasp a life preserver must certainly be assisted to do so. In what sense is the pumping action of an apparatus designed to facilitate absorption of the oxygen by the bloodstream any different from physically placing the life preserver around the waist of the drowning victim?

The commonly drawn distinction between "ordinary" and "extraordinary" means of treatment and the exclusion of "heroic" measures to preserve life have no parallel in Jewish sources. Indeed, one is hard-pressed to find appropriate terminology in rabbinic Hebrew to express such distinctions. They have entered contemporary moral discourse through the mediation of an entirely foreign religious tradition.

In discharging their responsibility with regard to prolongation of life, physicians must make use of any medical resources that are available. However, as shown elsewhere,[11] they are not obligated to employ procedures that are intrinsically hazardous and may shorten the life of the patient. Nor is either the physician or the patient obligated to employ a therapy that is experimental in nature.[12]

Palliation of Pain
Elimination of pain is assuredly a legitimate and laudable goal. According to some authorities, mitigation of pain is encompassed within the general obligation to heal.[13] Palliative treatment is certainly mandated by virtue of the commandment "and you shall love your neighbor as yourself" (Leviticus 19:18). When the dual goals of avoidance of pain and preservation of life come into conflict with one another, however, Judaism recognizes the paramount value and sanctity of life and, accordingly, assigns priority to preservation of life. Thus,

a number of authorities have expressly stated that nontreatment or withdrawal of treatment in order for the patient to be released from pain by death constitutes euthanasia and is not countenanced by Judaism.[14] This remains the case even if the patient pleads to be permitted to die. As stated by one prominent authority, "Even if the patient himself cries out, 'Let me be and do not give me any aid, because for me death is preferable,' everything possible must be done on behalf of the patient."[15]

Nevertheless, every prudent effort should be made to alleviate the patient's suffering. This includes aggressive treatment of pain even to a degree which at present is not common in medical practice. Physicians are reluctant to use morphine in high dosages because of the danger of depression of the cerebral center responsible for respiration. The effect of morphine administered in high doses is that the patient cannot control the muscles necessary for breathing. There is, however, no halakhic objection to providing such medication in order to control pain in the case of terminal patients even though palliation of pain may ultimately entail maintaining such a patient on a respirator. Similarly, there is no halakhic objection to the use of heroin in the control of pain in terminal patients. The danger of addiction under such circumstances is, of course, hardly a significant consideration. At present, the use of heroin is illegal even for medical purposes. Judaism affirms that everything in creation is designed for a purpose. Alleviation of otherwise intractable pain is a known beneficial use of heroin. Marijuana is effective in alleviating the nausea that is a side-effect of some forms of chemotherapy. There is every reason to believe that these drugs were given to man for the specific purpose of controlling pain and discomfort. Jewish teaching would enthusiastically endorse legislation legalizing the use – with adequate accompanying safeguards – of those substances in the treatment of terminal patients.

The basic principle that it is not obligatory to prolong the life of every patient is developed by Rabbi Mosheh Feinstein in *Iggerot Mosheh*, Hoshen Mishpat II, no. 73, sec. 1. In this responsum, *Iggerot Mosheh* cites the narrative recorded by the Gemara, Ketubbot 104b, describing the sickness and pain suffered by R. Judah the Prince. When R. Judah's maidservant saw that the prayers of his disciples did not effect either a cure or relief of his suffering, she successfully prayed for his death. *Iggerot Mosheh* concludes that in circumstances in which the physician has determined that the patient cannot be cured and that his or her life cannot be prolonged without concomitant suffering, further medication should not be administered. By the same token, Rabbi Feinstein declares that medications must be administered to alleviate pain provided that the medication does not shorten life even briefly. He also insists that oxygen be administered as needed, on the assumption that failure to administer oxygen will increase the suffering of the patient. In *Iggerot Mosheh*, Hoshen Mishpat ii, no. 74, sec. 1, Rabbi Feinstein again states that a cancer patient should be so informed if medication will merely prolong his life with suffering, and that such therapy should not be administered without the consent of the patient. In this responsum he emphasizes that sanctioning the withholding of therapy in cases of extreme pain should not be confused with decisions based upon "quality of life." *Iggerot Mosheh* emphatically declares that the life of a mentally incompetent person, and even of a patient in a permanent vegetative state, must be prolonged to the extent possible so long as the patient does not suffer extreme pain.

A similar pronouncement by the late Rabbi Shlomo Zalman Auerbach was published in *Halakhah u-Refu'ah*, ii (Jerusalem, 5741), 131, and reprinted with a minor linguistic change in his collected responsa, *Minkhat Shelomoh*, no. 91, sec. 24. The following is a literal translation of his statement:

> Many struggle with this question concerning treatment of a *goses*. Some are of the opinion that just as the Sabbath must be desecrated for ephemeral life (*hayyei sha'ah*), so is it similarly obligatory to compel the patient with regard to this, since he is not a proprietor with regard to himself [with the right] to relinquish even a single moment [of life]. However, it is reasonable that if the patient experiences great pain and suffering, or even extremely severe

psychological pain, [although] I think that it is mandatory to give him food[16] and oxygen for breathing even against his will, it is permissible to withhold medications that cause suffering to the patient[17] if the patient so demands. However, if the patient is God-fearing and is not mentally confused, it is extremely desirable to explain to him that a single hour of repentance in this world is more valuable than all of the world-to-come, as we find in tractate Sotah 20a that it is a "privilege" to suffer seven years rather than to die immediately.

Noteworthy is the fact that Rabbi Auerbach refers to two distinct situations, the case of a patient who steadfastly refuses treatment and the case of a patient who can be consulted with regard to his wishes, but ignores the situation of the incompetent patient who lacks decision-making capacity. Similarly, the earlier-cited statement, dated 29 Kislev 5755, speaks only of obligatory forms of treatment but fails to indicate whether, in the absence of an announced desire on the part of the patient, other forms of treatment are prohibited or whether they may be administered at the discretion of the family and/or physician. *Iggerot Mosheh* speaks of prolongation of the patient's pain as prohibited except with the patient's consent. Also noteworthy is Rabbi Auerbach's emphasis upon pain as a spiritual "benefit" or "privilege" and his strong recommendation that the patient be encouraged to accept prolongation of life to the extent medically possible despite the accompanying suffering.

Although the theory espoused by *Iggerot Mosheh* and Rabbi Auerbach is well founded, it seems to this writer that there is little room for its implementation. Their halakhic rulings proceed from the presumption that at least some patients must endure "great pain" or "suffering." While many patients undoubtedly do suffer unspeakable pain, that need not be the case. Recent medical literature is replete with articles and comments deploring the fact that physicians are inadequately trained in palliation of pain or are unwilling to utilize available means to control pain. In rejecting the patient's suffering of unrelieved pain as a valid motive for the practice of euthanasia, Dr. Porter Storey reports on his own treatment of some two thousand terminally ill patients and asserts that pain "can be effectively palliated by administering narcotic analgesics which can be used safely if the dose is carefully titrated against the symptoms."[18] Moreover, studies conducted over the past decade demonstrate that substantial and sustained doses of narcotics may be administered without risk to the patient.[19] An as yet unpublished report of the Bioethics Committee of the Montefiore Medical Center concludes that "The widespread belief that adequate pain control usually poses high risks of respiratory distress and a consequent hastening of death appears to be based more on long-standing myth than on medical fact." A manual published by the Washington Medical Association reports that "adequate interventions exist to control pain in 90–99% of patients."[20] The American Medical Association has stated that "the pain of most terminally ill patients can be controlled throughout the dying process without heavy sedation or anesthesia.... For a very few patients, however, sedation to a sleep-like state may be necessary in the last days or weeks of life to prevent the patient from experiencing severe pain."[21] From the vantage point of Halakhah, life-prolonging therapy may be withheld only to avoid excruciating pain. However, when pain can be controlled, the obligation to preserve and prolong life remains in full force.

A CONCLUDING COMMENT

A brief comment of the late Rabbi Yosef Eliyahu Henkin, of blessed memory, eloquently captures the Jewish attitude with regard to the emotionally charged issue of treatment of the terminally ill. Many years ago, when I first began to investigate issues of medical Halakhah, and when many now commonplace life-prolonging measures were still new, I off-handedly asked Rabbi Henkin, "How far is one obligated to go in order to prolong life?" Without the slightest hesitation he responded, *"Azoi lang vi a Yid ken leben, darf er velen leben"* ("So long as it is possible for a Jew to live, he ought to want to live").

Those words uttered by a blind, frail, saintly individual to whom life had clearly become a burden – but a sacred burden – made a profound impression upon me. That short, succinct statement reflects authentic Jewish values in a way that sometimes is submerged in learned responsa. Truly, sometimes one cannot see the forest because of the trees.

Notes and References

1. Arthur Hugh Clough, "The Latest Decalogue," in *The Oxford Book of Nineteenth-Century English Verse*, ed. John Hayward (Oxford, 1970), p. 609. These words, when quoted, are almost invariably cited in a literal sense. In actuality, the poet was not endorsing the moral position expressed in this couplet but was engaging in irony. See Maurice Strauss, *Familiar Medical Quotations* (Boston, 1968), p. 159b, n. 1.
2. This statement, of course, applies to life as defined by Halakhah. The status of a *nefel* (i.e., a nonviable neonate) requires independent analysis.
3. See *Shulhan Arukh*, Orah Hayyim 329:4.
4. See also *Tosefot Yom Tov*, Sotah 1:9.
5. See also R. Shlomo Yosef Zevin, *Le-Or ha-Halakhah*, 2nd ed. (Tel Aviv, 5717), pp. 318–335; cf. R. Sha'ul Israeli, in *Ha-Torah ve-ha-Medinah* 5–6 (5713–14): 106–111 and 7–8 (5715–17): 331–336. See also R. Simhah ha-Kohen Kook, in *Torah she-be-'al Peh* 13 (5736): 58–82.
6. It is clear that, when halakhically indicated, a patient is not only obligated to seek medical care but may be compelled to do so. See sources cited in J. David Bleich, "The Obligation to Heal in the Judaic Tradition: A Comparative Analysis," in *Jewish Bioethics*, ed. Fred Rosner and J. David Bleich (New York, 1979), p. 43, n. 100; cf. ibid., p. 42, n. 97. Since the obligation of rescue is phrased as a prohibition against standing idly by "the blood of your fellow," the source of an obligation to save one's own life is somewhat elusive. It is, of course, an uncontested halakhic principle that "A person is his own relative" (*adam karov ezel azmo*). See Sanhedrin 9b and 25a, Ketubbot 18b, and Yevamot 25b. By the same token, it may be argued that a person is his own "fellow" and thus owes himself the selfsame duties. See R. Zalman Nehemiah Goldberg, *Moriyyah* 8, nos. 3–4 (Elul 5738): 51, quoted in *Halakhah u-Refu'ah*, ed. R. Moshe Herschler, vol. 2 (Jerusalem, 5741), pp. 153–154; cf., however, R. Mordecai Jonah Rabinowitz, *Afikei Yam*, 11, no. 40; s.v. *ve-haya*. Note should also be taken of the fact that the Gemara, Bava Mezi'a 62a, cites the verse "and your brother shall live with you" (Leviticus 25:38) in establishing that preservation of one's own life must be given preference over the rescue of another. An obligation to preserve one's own life may readily be inferred from that definition. Also, Rambam, Hilkhot Roze'ah 11:4, cites the verse "take heed of yourself and safeguard yourself" (Deuteronomy 4:9) as establishing an obligation "to be watchful" with regard to any matter that poses a danger, as well as the negative commandment "And you shall not bring blood upon your house" (Deuteronomy 22:8) as establishing an obligation to remove a source of danger. See also Hilkhot Roze'ah 11:5. The latter verses serve to establish a positive command, whereas "nor shall you stand idly by the blood of your fellow" establishes a more stringent negative prohibition for failure to seek life-saving interventions.

Afikei Yam, II, no. 40, s.v. *ve-haya*, suggests that failure to preserve one's own life may be halakhically equivalent to suicide. *Pesikta Rabbati*, chap. 24, advances an exegetical rendition of *lo tirzah* (Exodus 20: 13) as *lo titrazah* in establishing that *felo-de-se* is encompassed in the prohibition against murder. See also *Halakhot Ketanot*, II, no. 231; *Bet Me'ir*, Yore De'ah 215:5; *Teshuvot Hatam Sofer*, Yore De'ah, no. 326; Mahari Perla, *Sefer ha-Mitzvot le-Rabbenu Sa'adia Ga'on*, mitzvot lo ta'aseh, no. 59; *Gesher ha-Hayyim*, I, chap. 25; and *Torah Shelemah*, Parashat Yitro, chap. 20, sec. 336. Rambam, Hilkhot Roze'ah 2:3, declares suicide to be prohibited on the basis of the verse "But your blood of your lives I will require" (Genesis 9:5). The ramifications of his citation of that verse are noted by *Minhat Hinnukh*, no. 34. Cf. Mahari Perla's comments on *Minhat Hinnukh*, ad loc. Cf. also R. Shimon Moshe Diskin, *Mas'et ha-Melekh* (Jerusalem, 5742), Hilkhot Roze'ah 2:3, reprinted in idem, *Mas'et ha-Melekh* (Jerusalem, 5749), IV, no. 433.

In point of fact, *Afikei Yam*'s position that the obligation to seek a cure for a life-threatening illness and to take other necessary measures to prolong one's own life is based upon the prohibition against suicide may be inferred from the comments of Ran, Shevu'ot 28a. Rambam, Hilkhot Shevu'ot 5:20, rules that one who swears not to eat for seven days has sworn a vain oath and, accordingly, is to be punished immediately for that infraction but may eat whenever he wishes. Ran agrees with Rambam's ruling but not with his reasoning. Rambam regards the oath as vain because it cannot be fulfilled, just as an oath not to sleep for a period of three days is not capable of fulfillment. Ran disagrees and argues that a person cannot keep himself awake but can refrain from eating even though he endangers himself in the process. Nevertheless, Ran regards the oath as vain because "one who has sworn to kill himself has actually sworn to transgress the words of the Torah, for Scripture states explicitly 'But your blood of your lives will I require'...or also 'take heed of yourself and safeguard yourself.'" Ran explicitly declares that the prohibition against suicide and the obligation to avoid danger mandate active intervention to seek food in order to sustain life. The selfsame obligations require the individual to seek medical treatment.

7. *Yated Ne'eman*, 29 Kislev 5755, p. 56. See also *Yated ha-Shavu'ah*, 19 Tevet 5755, p. 9.
8. *Shulhan Arukh*, Yoreh De' ah 339:1.
9. Ibid.
10. Shabbat 151b and Semahot 1:4.
11. See J. David Bleich, *Jewish Bioethics*, pp. 29–33; and idem, *Judaism and Healing* (New York, 1981), pp. 119–121.
12. See *Jewish Bioethics*, p. 28; *Judaism and Healing*, pp. 116–118; and the more extensive discussion in J. David Bleich, *Contemporary Halakhic Problems*, vol. 4 (New York, 1995), pp. 203–217.
13. See *Tzitz Eliezer*, XIII, no. 87. See also R. Nathan Zevi Friedman, in *Ha-Torah ve-ha-Medinah* 5–6, p. 229; and R. Iser Y. Unterman, in *Torah she-be-'al Peh* 11 (5729): 14.
14. Cf., however, R. Isaac Liebes, *Teshuvot Bet Avi*, II, no. 153, p. 213. Rabbi Liebes cites Rambam's comment in his *Commentary on the Mishnah*, Nedarim 4:4 (see also idem, *Mishneh Torah*, Hilkhot Nedarim 6:8) indicating that the scriptural exhortation with regard to returning lost property also serves to establish an obligation requiring the physician to render professional services in life-threatening situations. See Sanhedrin 73a. Rabbi Liebes comments that "on the basis of this derivation, the physician is obligated to restore [the patient's] body, i.e., in a situation in which there is hope to restore the body entirely, but in a situation in which by means of this [treatment] he will no longer restore

[the patient's] body, but, on the contrary, will cause him additional pain and suffering, with regard to this he is not at all obligated." Rabbi Liebes's argument is not compelling for two reasons: (1) The Gemara, Sanhedrin 73a, applies this obligation to situations involving a person drowning in a river, being mauled by a wild animal, and under attack by armed robbers. The "loss" to be restored is life per se, not health or well-being. The obligation to restore property is in no way related to the duration of the useful life of the lost item. Thus restoration of the body should be required regardless of the fact that longevity anticipation is limited to a brief period of time. (2) Although, as indicated by the Gemara, Bava Kama 85a, specific scriptural authorization is required to treat the sick, once such sanction has been granted, the obligation with regard to therapeutic intervention is no different from other forms of preservation of life. Failure to intervene constitutes a violation of the commandment "nor shall you stand idly by the blood of your fellow" (Leviticus 19:16). Thus *Shulhan Arukh*, Yoreh De'ah 336:1, states: "The Torah gave permission to the physician to heal. This is a religious precept and is included in the category of saving life, and if the physician withholds [his services] it is considered as shedding blood." Nontherapeutic rescue, as described in Sanhedrin 73a (e.g., rescue from drowning or from a wild animal), is mandatory regardless of age, state of health, or length of the natural longevity anticipation of the victim. Accordingly, equating medical intervention with other forms of rescue serves to establish an obligation to prolong life even if a complete cure is not possible. See *Perishah*, Yore De'ah 336:4; *Ramat Rahel*, no. 21; and *Tzitz Eliezer*, 11, no. 25, chap. 7. Cf. *Iggerot Mosheh*, Hoshen Mishpat, 11, no. 74, see. 1, s.v. *ve-pashut*. Moreover, the rescuer's monetary obligation is derived from Leviticus 19:6, which establishes an obligation for payment of medical expenses in cases of battery and clearly applies even when a complete cure is impossible.

15. *Tzitz Eli'ezer*, IX, no. 47, sec. 5.
16. Cf. *Teshuvot Bet Avi*, 11, no. 153, s.v. *u-le-dina* and *sikkum*.
17. There is perhaps some ambiguity with regard to the implication of this statement. The phrase "it is permissible to withhold medications that cause suffering" standing alone, might be understood as limited to suffering caused by the medication, i.e., as a side-effect rather than by the underlying condition. However, the earlier reference to a patient who "experiences great pain and suffering" seems to indicate that the suffering to which reference is made is not the product of the medication but of the underlying pathology. Moreover, there does not appear to be any halakhic consideration that would support such a distinction between pain that is the result of a malady and pain induced by medication. Indeed, no distinction of that nature appears in the statement of 29 Kislev 5755 to which Rabbi Auerbach was a signatory.
18. Porter Storey, "It's Over, Debbie" (letter), *Journal of the American Medical Association* 259, no. 14 (April 8, 1988): 2095.
19. See T.D. Walsh, "Opiates and Respiratory Function in Advanced Cancer," *Recent Results in Cancer Research* 39 (1984): 1115–1117; E. Bruera et al., "Effects of Morphine on the Dyspnea of Terminal Cancer Patients," *Journal of Pain and Symptom Management* 5, no. 6 (December 1990): 341–344; M. Angel, "The Quality of Mercy" (editorial), *New England Journal of Medicine* 306, no. 2 (January 14, 1982): 98–99. See also R.R. Miller and H. Jick, "Clinical Effects of Meperidine in Hospitalized Medical Patients," *Journal of Clinical Pharmacology* 18, no. 4 (April 1978): 180–189; R.R. Miller, "Analgesics," in *Drug Effects in Hospitalized Patients*, ed. R. Miller and D.J. Greenblatt (New York, 1976), pp. 133–164.

---

20. Albert Einstein, "Overview of Cancer Pain Management," in *Pain Management and Care of the Terminal Patient*, ed. Judy Kornell (<<**town?**>>: Rabbi Bleich's answer: There is no town given in the book). Washington State Medical Association, 1992), p. 4. Another study indicates that when treated by skilled practitioners, the pain of 98 percent of patients in hospice care can be relieved. See American Medical Association Council on Scientific Affairs, "Good Care of the Dying Patient," *Journal of the American Medical Association* 275, no. 6 (February 14, 1996): 475. See also C.S. Cleeland et al., "Pain and Its Treatment in Outpatients with Metastatic Cancer," *New England Journal of Medicine* 330, no. 9 (March 3, 1994): 592.

21. Brief of the American Medical Association et al., as *amici curiae* in support of petitioners, at 6, *Washington v. Glucksberg*, 117 S. Ct. 2258 (1997) (No. 96–110).

"Some" Reflections on Jewish Tradition and the End-of-Life Patient

Leonard S. Kravitz

I BEGIN with a necessary digression: a remembrance from a freshman college course in logic. "All men are mortal, Socrates is a man, and therefore Socrates is mortal." In that course, I learned that the key element in the proposition was the word "all" in the first sentence; it includes Socrates and thus leads to the conclusion that Socrates is mortal. Had the sentence begun with the word "some," we would not know whether Socrates was included in some, for if only some are mortal, it may be that some are not, and thus we would not know whether Socrates is mortal. To establish the mortality of Socrates would then require further argumentation; we would have to look at Socrates as a specific case, and we would not be helped by the less than universal statement that some men are mortal.

This digression is necessary if we are to deal with statements about Jewish ethics and caring for the end-of-life patient. These statements, as we shall see, are essentially "some" statements, whether they deal with "Jewish," "ethics," "caring," or "end of life"; that is to say, they present a selection of notions from a larger group, all the while claiming that they present the totality of the group. Beginning with the word "Jewish" will clarify the issue: To what does it refer? A group of people who identify as Jews or a literature associated with that group? If it refers to the group, does it assume that all members of the group agree? Does it assume that those members of the group who conceive of themselves as "religious" agree on the meaning and expectations of a religious commitment? Even were we to say that "Jewish" "refers to those individuals who consciously govern their lives by the tenets of their faith,"[1] we could not be certain that agreement might be found as to the content and meaning of the phrase "the tenets of…faith" among the various parties in Judaism, nor even among those who might be designated as Orthodox in their belief. The term "Jewish," therefore, refers to the positions of "some" Jews, among whom are to be found those who deem themselves religious Jews and also those who do not. Even among religious Jews, there is no agreement as to the content of the term, for in the modem world, there are different forms of Jewish religiosity, and with that, different approaches to particular problems. Thus unanimity of outlook is not to be found among religious Jews. Thus their views are "some" views in the same manner as the views of those who view themselves as secular Jews. It follows, then, that if "some" Jews hold a particular position, it may be that "some" Jews do not. Thus no Jewish position can be derived from an "all" statement, and each Jewish position will have to present an independent argument to be accepted.

The ethics part of "Jewish ethics" will be even more problematic. "Ethics" bespeaks universal notions, and thus we shall hear that Jewish ethics champions "the sanctity/inviolability of life."[2] On the basis of such a view, some would hold that any interference with the end-of-life patient is tantamount to, and indeed is, murder.[3] If we reflect on these two conjoined notions, that life is sacred and that interference with life, even life that is terminal, constitutes murder, we face the problem of "all" and "some." However we may conceive of the sanctity of life, we know that Judaism is not a pacifist tradition. The Bible is filled with accounts of war,[4] and rabbinic tradition accepted war.[5] The rabbis distinguished between obligatory and voluntary wars; the former were wars against the Seven Nations that inhabited the Land, battles against Amalek, and wars in defense of Israelite cities; the latter were wars waged to extend the boundaries of the Land.

War of whatever kind entails the destruction of life, not only, as we have seen in our time, of combatants, but also of noncombatants (our age has hidden the latter reality under the term "collateral damage"). But if war with its concomitant killing is acceptable, the notion of sanctity of life is reduced to a kind of "some" statement: some kind of life is sacrosanct, but not all. But if only some life is sacrosanct, we will have to establish why that life is sacrosanct and other kinds of life are not. It will not help to refer to a theological notion of the human person *be-tzelem Elohim*, "in the image of God," if such a description does not cover everyone, including one's enemies. Moreover, as the history of warfare indicates, one's enemies today may be one's friends tomorrow, just as one's friends today may well be one's enemies tomorrow.

Not only does Judaism accept war, it accepts capital punishment as a means of dealing with internal enemies who are thought to threaten the physical or moral status of Jewish or general society. Not only do we read biblical passages enjoining the death penalty, but we read passages describing it being carried out for transgressions which to the modern eye do not seem worthy of death.[6] The rabbis prescribed four methods of capital punishment,[7] and medieval Jews carried out executions.[8] But capital punishment, like war, makes any statement about the "sanctity of life" a "some" statement. Just as the lives of one's external enemies are excluded from being considered sacrosanct, so are the lives of one's internal enemies.

If one accepts killing as licit when carried out in war, even in wars not fought in self-defense, and if one accepts killing as licit as a means of dealing with criminals, a means which is not ipso facto necessary, since there are other means, such as life imprisonment, to deal with those who commit horrendous acts, one is hard put to define "murder." The dictionary's definition, "the unlawful and intentional killing of one human being by another,"[9] does help much because it depends on the definition of "unlawful"; one may ask who defines what is lawful and what is unlawful. One should remember that the Nuremberg Laws were *laws*! One might argue that the Nazi murder of Jews was both lawful and intentional! A cynic reflecting on war and on capital punishment might argue that murder is that which is proscribed to the individual but permitted to a government.

On further reflection, one might wonder that if one can kill innocent people in war (collateral damage) and guilty people in peace (capital punishment) and yet not call such acts murder, how can one call aiding a suffering and terminal patient to meet death murder? One might argue that murder is the act of killing an unwilling victim; but then such a definition would fit killing in war and killing as an act of capital punishment. Enabling a suffering person who has no prospect of recovering to reach the death that already beckons is hardly an act performed on an unwilling victim.

Strangely enough, a talmudic discussion of capital punishment provides insight into the issue of euthanasia.[10] According to the sage Rabbah bar Abbahu, one should procure for the condemned criminal a *mitah yafah,* a "nice death," and thus fulfill the biblical commandment "Thou shall love thy neighbor as thyself"![11] And what is a "nice death"? The commentator Rashi tells us: *she-yamut maher* – "that he should die quickly."[12] A nice death is to die quickly; to die slowly, we may deduce, is to die an ugly death. For the condemned, to die quickly is to suffer less; to die slowly is to suffer more.

It is the connection between suffering and time that brings us to the issue of euthanasia. Were the dying person not suffering but perfectly comfortable and in possession of his or her faculties, the issue would never arise. Every person, every day at every moment moves toward the grave; if life were free of pain and full of delight, who would wish to speed the journey? One thinks of euthanasia only when a person is dying and suffering and there seems no way of staving off the first condition and palliating the second. Thus euthanasia entails two elements: death which is imminent and pain which cannot be controlled.

What should the physician do? The medical profession is committed to care for the patient. Yet what does "caring" mean in this context? Clearly, if the physician can heal the patient, then healing is what the physician should do; if palliating the pain is possible, then palliation is what the physician should do. Alas, in some cases the physician can do neither; it is at this point that we have the problem with "caring." What does it mean in this context? There seems to be no trade-off: the patient's suffering will not lead to recovery and the patient's suffering cannot be controlled. The physician can neither heal nor remove pain; what, then, should the physician do? One possibility is to do nothing – to not act at all; but the patient will continue to suffer. Is allowing a moribund patient to suffer caring for the patient in any sense of the word "care"?

If the physician is unable to cure and unable to palliate but cares about the patient, and wishes to care for the patient, what then should the physician do? If a failing life can be extended but not without pain, would it not occur to the physician that such a life should not be extended? Rashi's explanation of *mitah yafah* comes to mind – that the patient be enabled *she-yamut maher* (i.e., to die quickly).

A physician who set out to to ascertain the Jewish attitude to euthanasia might read the following statement by a Reform rabbi:

> It is a curious, but incontrovertible fact that the theory of euthanasia, even in its most restricted construction, has never invaded Jewish thought.... The Jewish ideal of the sanctity of human life...would suffer incalculable harm if...men were at liberty to determine the conditions under which they might make an end to their own lives and the lives of other men.[13]

The physician might also read this statement by an ordained Orthodox rabbi who is a practicing physician:

> The practice of euthanasia – whether active or passive – is contrary to the teachings of Judaism. Any positive act designed to hasten the death of the patient is equated with murder in Jewish law.... No matter how laudable the intentions of the person performing the act of mercy-killing may be, his deed constitutes an act of homicide.... Only the Creator, who bestows the gift of life, may relieve man of that life, even when it has become a burden rather than a blessing.[14]

With such expressed certainty as to the "Jewish" view of euthanasia, one might have expected a plethora of textual bases for this view. In truth there are few. There is a text in the Mishnah which warns that one should not close the eyes of a dying person,[15] and the explanation in the Gemara that doing so would be like touching the dying flame of a candle and thereby immediately extinguishing it.[16] Closing the eyes of the dying person hastens that person's death; to do so is to be a *shofekh damim* "one who sheds blood." There are two talmudic texts commonly adduced as the basis, by way of interpretation, of the so-called Jewish view of euthanasia.[17] There is a passage in the Midrash which on reflection raises substantial questions about this view. There is a passage in the Gemara that defines what is meant by a moribund patient, and there is a passage in a post-talmudic tractate which echoes the Mishnah and Gemara texts quoted above, and there is a reflection on that passage in a commentary on the *Shulhan Arukh*.

Just as we have noted, in discussing the acceptance of war and capital punishment, that there is a lack of unanimity in Jewish sources on what constitutes being a *shofekh damim*, "one who sheds blood," so too we shall discover that there is no unanimity on the acceptability of euthanasia. Indeed, a close reading of the two talmudic texts will suggest that they support the reverse of the ideas others attribute to them.

The talmudic texts and the midrashic passage present events in the lives of three tannaim: Hananiah ben Teradyon, Judah the Prince, and Yose (Ha-Galili) ben Halafta, who lived in the second and third centuries C.E.[18] If we follow the presumptive order of the tannaim mentioned, the two talmudic texts contain an account of the execution of Hananiah and an account of the last days of Judah the Prince. The midrashic passage depicts an event in the life of Yose. As important as the three sages were, more important for our purposes are the other figures who appear in these stories. These figures we shall characterize as the kind executioner, the troubled maid, and the surprising old lady.

The first text is often quoted as the exemplar of the Jewish view of euthanasia. Having condemned Hananiah for the crime of teaching Torah, the Romans decided to make an example of him by burning him alive. They unrolled scrolls of the Torah, wrapped the parchment around him, surrounded him with cut tree boughs, and then ignited the parchment and the wood. To keep the fire from killing him too quickly, so that he would suffer longer, the Romans tied wet mats of wool around his body. As the Talmud continues the story:

> Rabbi [Hananiah ben] Teradyon's students said to him: "Rabbi…
> open your mouth that the fire may enter [and you die]." He said
> to them, "It is better that He who gave my soul should take it and
> let no one harm himself." The executioner asked him, "Rabbi, if I
> make the fire hotter and remove the mats from your body, will you
> bring me into the World to Come?" He answered, "Yes." "Swear
> to me!" [said the executioner]. He [the executioner] immediately
> removed the mats and increased the flames. His [Hananiah's] soul
> speedily departed. Then he [the executioner] leaped up and fell
> into the fire. A *bat kol* went out and proclaimed: "Rabbi Hananiah
> and the executioner are prepared for the Life to Come." Rabbi
> [Judah the Prince] wept and said, "Some may attain their world
> in [but] one moment, while others may take many years."[19]

Rabbi Hananiah's response that "It is better that He who gave my soul should take it and let no one harm himself" has been taken as teaching that only God should end life[20] and that no one should intrude in the dying process.[21]

But does the story teach that? When one looks at it again, one may derive a far different lesson. The story does not present a consistent position. Since it purports to describe events occurring over time, the story suggests that Rabbi Hananiah's immense suffering led him to change his mind and facilitate his own death! As given in the story, the kindly executioner's question was more than a request for information; it was a proposal of a contract. That the executioner asked the rabbi to swear to his answer indicates that both executioner and rabbi knew what was to be the outcome and what was to be the consideration, the quid pro quo.[22]

To attempt to force consistency in the story, one would have to have the rabbi remain silent or have him reply to the executioner, "If you are asking for information, that is one thing, but if you are asking for my concurrence, that is another, for I will remain constant in position and consistent with my earlier statement, and therefore will do nothing which might in any way speed my death."

But the story does not have Rabbi Hananiah remain silent, nor does it have him say what I have suggested he might have said. It would have been inhuman to expect him to follow either alternative. It is human, understandable, and, indeed, to be expected that Hananiah acted as he did; faced by certain death and experiencing terrible pain, he sought to avoid the latter by accelerating the former.

Acceleration of the dying process and an attempt to derail that process form the contrasting elements in the story of the death of Rabbi Judah the Prince. When he became very ill and was facing death, the sages sought to save him by proclaiming a fast and making an appeal for Divine mercy. Moreover, said they, if anyone lets it be known that Rabbi is dying, that person should be stabbed with a sword.

The story continues with the actions of Rabbi's troubled maid:

> The maid of Rabbi went up to the roof. She said, "Those on high are seeking Rabbi, and those below are seeking Rabbi. [Those 'on high' are the Divine and angelic powers seeking Rabbi's death; 'those below" are his students, praying that he will live.] May it be God's will that those below conquer those on high!" [But] when she saw how many times he would enter the privy and how he was suffering, she said, "Would that those on high win against those below." The rabbis [however] did not cease imploring God's mercy. She then took a vase and threw it from the roof. They [the rabbis] were interrupted in their prayer [lit., they were silenced in their requesting God's mercy], and Rabbi's soul departed.[23]

What the troubled maid did relates to the assumptions of the story: prayer was believed to be a mechanism that could either maintain or end the life of Rabbi. By throwing the vase from the roof, the maid disrupted the mechanism. Hers was a physical act; she took a vase and threw it.[24] The sound the vase made as it smashed onto the ground startled the students, stopping their prayer, and Rabbi died. One may say that the maid's action enabled Rabbi to die, or one may say that her action caused him to die; in either case, her act precipitated his death. She acted; he died!

There are some troubling aspects to the story. The troubled maid acted without reference to the wishes of the old man. She did not ask him about the intensity of his pain, but deduced it by observing his actions. One might worry that this story could be used to derive the notion that euthanasia can be applied without consent, and that pain can be determined merely by observation – and by someone who is not a medical professional at that! After all, nowhere is the maid condemned for what she did.[25] We mention this not to condemn the lady but to indicate how difficult it is to deduce principles, whether universal (the "all" kind) or general (the "some" kind), from such stories.

Although Rabbi, according to the story, did not request his own death, there is a rabbinic text which tells of a person requesting and receiving advice about ending his life. Unlike Rabbi Hananiah or Rabbi Judah the Prince, the person in this story is not in great pain; rather she is described as suffering from ennui. In this story too, prayer is a life-maintaining mechanism. We read:

> There is a story of a woman who grew very old. She came before Rabbi Yose [Ha-Galili] ben Halafta. She said to him, "Rabbi, I have become too old. Life is repugnant to me. I can taste neither food nor drink. I would like to depart from this world." He said to her, "How is it that you have lived so long?" She answered, "Every day I go early to the synagogue, even if in doing so I have to stop [doing] something I like." He said to her, "For three days in a row, stop going to the synagogue!" This she did. On the third day, she became ill and died.[26]

We should reflect that the sage to whom this surprising old lady went did not upbraid her, nor did he proclaim to her Judaism's supposed opposition to euthanasia. He simply asked her how she had lived so long. Hearing her answer, he devised a plan by which she might bring her life to an end. If anything, the story as it stands gives an example of the acceptance of euthanasia; and note that euthanasia was requested in this instance not because of the suffering caused by pain, but because of the distress caused by the physical resultants of old age.

In both the story of the troubled maid and the story of the surprising old lady, prayer is held to be a life-maintaining mechanism and interrupting or ceasing prayer becomes the means of ending life. The troubled maid prays initially for Rabbi to live; then, seeing his suffering, she stops praying, and finally, by throwing the vase, she interrupts the prayers of Rabbi's students. The surprising old lady is instructed to cease praying so that her life may end; she does and she dies.

Time plays a role in both stories: at first everyone, including Rabbi's maid, wants Rabbi to live; then time passes and the maid no longer wishes that he live; more time passes, and following the maid's action, Rabbi ceases living. For the old lady, passing through time has changed her view of life; she no longer wishes to live. Going to Rabbi Yose, she receives advice about what to do on three successive days: if she does not go to the synagogue and does not pray, she will be dead. Go she does not, and die she does. From the assumptions of the story, had the lady changed her mind on the third day and gone to the synagogue to pray, she would have lived.

The last story, about the old lady who asked, the second story, about the maid who acted, and even the first story, about the kind executioner who contracted, belie any notion that Judaism has always opposed euthanasia. Indeed, the disparity between what is claimed to be the position of Judaism and the plain sense of the texts upon which this position is supposedly based makes the reader who approaches the texts without presuppositions wonder how the notion that Judaism opposes euthanasia ever came about. The three different stories, on reflection, remind of us of Rashi's definition of a *mitah yafah*, or "nice death" – *she-yamut maher* "that one dies quickly," that is to say, quicker than one might die otherwise.

The three rabbinic texts discussed above, two talmudic and one midrashic, provide no basis for opposing euthanasia and, indeed, can be read as allowing it. In addition, there is a post-talmudic text, Semahot, which provides more of a basis for opposing euthanasia. However, we must first turn to a passage in the Gemara that deals with the *goses*, or moribund patient, whose status has certain legal consequences. This passage defines the *goses* (dying patient) in contradistinction to the *holeh* (the ordinary sick patient), stating "and [as for] the *holeh*, the majority of them live, and [as for] the *goses*, the majority of them die.[27]

That the *goses* presents a "some" situation rather than an "all" situation, since only a "majority" of moribund patients will die but not all, may have provided some protection for the minority; members of the minority may live if nothing deleterious is done to them. This will enable us to understand what we shall read in Semahot. The passage says that the *goses*

> is regarded as a living entity in respect to all matters of the world.... We do not tie up his cheekbones, or stop up his apertures, or place a metal vessel or anything that chills on his navel, as it is stated, "Before the silver cord is snapped asunder and the golden bowl is shattered, and the pitcher broken is at the fountain" (Eccles.12:6).... We may not move him, or place him on sand or salt until he dies.... We may not close the eyes of a dying man. Whoever touches or moves him is a murderer. For [as] Rabbi Meir used to say, "He can be compared to a lamp which is dripping. Should a man touch it, he extinguishes it. Similarly, whosoever closes the eyes of a dying man is considered to have taken his life."[28]

One might argue that since it is not absolutely certain that the *goses* will die on his own, any interference might push him (or her) over from life to death. Thus moving or touching the patient is forbidden. One may do nothing to bring death quicker. What if there were something that delayed death? If one may not speed the departure of the soul, may one remove an impediment to its departure? According to Moses Isserles (1525–1572), also known as the Ramah,

...if there is anything which causes a hindrance to the departure of the soul, such as the presence near the patient's house of a knocking noise, such as wood chopping, or if there is salt on the patient's tongue, and these hinder the soul's departure, it is permissible to remove them from there because no act is involved with this at all but only the removal of the impediment.[29]

The passage from Semahot and the comment by the Ramah have been taken as indicating the difference between active and passive euthanasia.[30] Although the first passage prohibits any action which would bring death quicker, the later comment permits actions which do. A moment's reflection precludes us from accepting the Ramah's statement that "no act is involved" in the activities described. To stop the sound of wood being chopped, one must go to the wood chopper and tell him to stop; to remove the salt from the patient's tongue, one must reach into the patient's mouth to remove it. It should be clear that we are not entering into the question of whether in fact rhythmic sounds or salt on the tongue prolong life; we simply note that stopping the former and removing the latter are actions done and not actions refrained from being done.

It is here that the notion that there is a difference between active and passive euthanasia becomes muddled and most unclear. If, at this moment, the sounds and the salt are keeping the patient alive, then stopping the one and removing the other are, depending on one's personal sensibility, either allowing the patient to die or killing the patient. Just as the troubled maid dropped the vase and thereby interrupted the process of prayer that was keeping Rabbi alive, so stopping the wood chopper's rhythmic sounds would interrupt a process that was keeping a patient alive, and similarly, removing the salt would interrupt the process of its dissolution which was keeping a patient alive. In these three cases of interfering with a process, one person acted and another person died. It is hard to see a metaphysical difference between these cases, even if one thought that the first was an example of active euthanasia and the last two of passive euthanasia. In all three cases, the person who acted intended the outcome. In the three cases, that which was intended, the death of the patient, occurred.

One wonders how stopping the rhythmic sound or removing the salt would be different, in essence, from disconnecting a moribund patient's oxygen line. In each of the above cases, there is an interruption of a process. The example of the oxygen line, however, suggests how the advance of technology has made the distinction between active and passive euthanasia exceedingly dubious. In the past, not bringing a cylinder of oxygen into the hospital room of a dying patient suffering intractable pain might have been called an act of passive euthanasia. Nowadays, in every modern hospital, there is an oxygen line in the wall of the room; one need not bring in a cylinder, the oxygen is already there. One can disconnect the patient from the already existing line for the same reason as one might in the past have not brought in the oxygen cylinder.

Thus modern technology has obviated the distinction between active and passive euthanasia, making it a distinction without a difference. But modern technology has created the problem to which the quandary of euthanasia is here addressed. The *goses* of old was only expected to live for three days.[31] Modern technology can extend the dying process for far more than three days. One might suspect that the modem term "euthanasia" would never have arisen were the patient, whatever the degree of suffering, to live and suffer for only three days.[32] Modern technology can enable the patient to live for more than three days and, alas, suffer for more than three days, since it can deal with some pain but not all pain, and not some pain for an extended period. What should be done? According to some, do nothing![33] But in truth, something is being done, if only to keep the patient alive. To do nothing is to allow the patient to suffer, not because there is a hope of recovery, but because we are unwilling to do something or perhaps because we think that suffering (for someone else, one must honestly admit) is preferable to death.[34]

What if the patient were to say, "I would rather die than undergo any more of this unbearable suffering" – what then? Some hold that one should pay no attention to such a statement, and that "every-thing possible should be done on behalf of the patient."[35] "On behalf of the patient," one wonders? How can purposeless suffering be "on behalf of the patient"? Only, perhaps, if one holds that the patient by such suffering gains approbation through proving some point, such as "dignity in the face of death"![36]

But to treat an unwilling patient or to have an unwilling patient demonstrate some abstract virtue is deny that patient the most basic right of a human being, the right to be left alone. The contract the patient makes with the physician assumes that the patient ultimately decides what is to be done with and to him/her, otherwise the physi-cian could do to the patient whatever the physician thinks ought to be done. To exaggerate the issue so as to clarify it, if a patient, say, came to a physician to have a broken arm set, and the physician thought that the patient also needed the repair of a hernia, the patient would have no recourse if the physician performed the operation by force and without obtaining the patient's consent. Neither a physician's of-fice nor a hospital is a prison; the patient can always walk out, albeit "against medical advice." If this is true for a comparatively healthy pa-tient, it should be true for an end-of-life patient.

A physician who would be unwilling to cease treatment regard-less of the wishes of the patient should so inform the patient before beginning treatment, whether the patient is comparatively healthy or an end-of-life patient. I would not wish to be the patient of such a physician whatever the state of my health.

The issue, then, is less than the theoretical issue of the autonomy of the human being vis-à-vis the Divine. It is less because it deals sim-ply with the contractual relationship between physician and patient. The question of whether one has the right to dispose of one's own body, the argument that "man is but a custodian of his body – bound by the ground rules imposed on him by the Creator and ultimate owner of his body – the Almighty,"[37] seems to be forgotten when the trumpets of war are blown or when a scaffold is erected. If war and capital punishment trump the claim of sanctity of life, they trump as well the notion that human beings are but the custodians of their bodies unable to act upon them in any lethal way. If one can act in a lethal way on another person's body, even against that person's will, it is hard to argue that one may not act willingly against one's own body! Yes, that would be suicide. But suicide has been reported in Jewish tradition, although often disguised as something else. How else describe the death of Samson? "Let me die with the Philistines," said he.[38] It was a conscious act on his part, associated with revenge against his tormentors. We have the case of Saul. Badly wounded, he first asked his armor-bearer, "Draw thy sword and thrust me through," and when the armor-bearer refused, he fell upon his sword. His recalcitrant armor-bearer then fell on his own sword and died.[39] There is the mass suicide of the four hundred boys and girls being taken to Rome for a life of "shame," forced prostitution, who threw themselves into the sea.[40] It should be noted that what the unfortunate children anticipated had not yet happened; they committed suicide not because of what they were currently experiencing but because of what they feared they might in future experience. That the Gemara adds the biblical verse "Yea, for Thy sake we are killed all the day long; we are counted as sheep to the slaughter"[41] suggests that their act of suicide was not condemned, but lauded.

Another way one may view these tragic children is as martyrs and Judaism has long accepted martyrdom; but martyrdom is, after all, suicide for a higher purpose. Martyrdom and and the preceding examples of suicide make any statement that Judaism totally opposes suicide a "some" statement. That being the case, every instance of suicide has to be judged on its own, not in the sense that one can second guess why a person committed suicide, but because in some cases taking one's own life might be understandable and perhaps acceptable. A responsum written by a Reform rabbi dealing with a woman suffering from Huntington's disease presents Judaism's opposition to suicide as an "all" statement, but nonetheless displays an empathetic understanding of suicide as a possible option.

> The path of this disease is clearly known and the degenerative effects are terrible, both for the individual involved and those dear

to her.... [While] we can empathize with her wish to commit suicide, it would be difficult for us to approve of this act as Judaism
has and continues to object strongly to suicide. The problems
which arise under slightly different conditions with other diseases
or other circumstances do not make it possible for us to assent to
her wish, but we understand it.[42]

Note that it was other cases, "other diseases or other circumstances,"
that precluded the acceptance of suicide in the particular case of
Huntington's disease. Thus it was a fear that acceptance of suicide
would be universalized that precluded the acceptance of suicide in this
specific case. Yet if there were universalization in the other direction,
that is to say, no absolute rejection of suicide, then each case of possible suicide could be judged on a case-by-case basis. The final judgment, like many other judgments that rational people make, would
be made on a gain-loss pattern. Such a judgment would be and could
be made only by the person contemplating the act. Surely, the gain
of life would offset anything but the most dire of situations; the loss
of life would only make sense were life ending and filled with intractable pain. Suicide, defined by the dictionary as "the act of an instance
of taking one's own life voluntarily and intentionally, esp. by a person of years of discretion and sound mind,"[43] may present different
problems for the end-of-life patient. There are such questions as the
means of taking one's life, the status and location of the patient, and
the enactments of the civil law. Depending on the definition, refusing
food or hydration may be suicide, a refusal to take certain drugs or
the taking of other drugs may be viewed as suicide, to say nothing of
the use of a knife or a firearm. If suicide is accomplished "voluntarily
and intentionally," then it follows that the patient must be conscious
to accomplish it. What if the patient drifts in and out of consciousness? What if the patient is unconscious but left a written instrument
detailing the conditions under which no further treatment should be
applied and no food or water be given, and those conditions are met?
What if the patient is conscious but physically unable to accomplish
the act – can someone else help? Does help mean providing the drugs

and putting them in the near vicinity of the patient? Does it mean injecting the fatal drug? What is the responsibility of the physician to carry out the wishes of the patient?

Inasmuch as under certain circumstances suicide is both understandable and acceptable, it would seem that a patient's conscious refusal to take food or hydration could be accompanied by the physician's prescribing of sedatives to prevent discomfort. Perhaps the physician could also provide, in the sense of placing them near at hand, the drugs that might enable the patient to end life. Whether a physician might inject other drugs to facilitate the patient's death would depend on the physician's conscience and the civil law, but one suspects that physicians have being doing this for some time.

Very often it is not the physician who is asked to facilitate suicide but a member of the family or a close friend. That very closeness may create a problem for the patient and for the family members or a friend. If, for example, a patient suffering with Huntington's disease is not able to accomplish her own demise and turns to a member of her family or a close friend to help her do what she cannot do alone, that family member or friend now has an interest in the patient's death. The friend or family member cannot act in a disinterested manner, perhaps for the best of motives, in that the death of the sufferer will free him or her from the distress of observing the patient's pain. Or perhaps for less good motives, such as the monetary benefit to the family member in that the patient will no longer need to be treated. For the best and worst of reasons, it would seem that involving a family member or a friend may not be a good choice. The attending physician would be the better choice.

The problem of dealing with the end-of-life-patient is aggravated in the case of patients who are unconscious and unable to convey their wishes. Where patients have left instructions as to their care at the end of life, the burden of benefit is taken from the shoulders of their family members or friends, who can then attempt to carry out the instructions as far as they are able and the law allows. A concerned relative or friend can convey the patient's instructions to the attending physician if the patient has not already done so. The best assistance a relative or friend can confer to both the patient and the physician is to serve as witness to the intentions of the patient.

What of patients who are unconscious but never left instructions about their terminal care? Such cases present a more difficult situation. Replaying the role of Rabbi's concerned maid – that is, bringing about death without regard to the will of the patient – presents moral and legal problems. An unconscious patient is presumably free of pain. As discussed above, it is pain, implacable pain, untreatable pain, which is the major consideration for speeding the end of life, and this consideration does not here exist. Moreover, if one holds that one owns one's own life, then only those who are conscious can decide to end their lives. Therefore, it would be difficult to justify any action by an onlooker.

But such a judgment has an impact on the series of questions raised by the issue of disconnecting the respirator of different patients in different physical states. The simplest case is that of the patient who has suffered brain death and whose bodily functions are being maintained by the respirator. Since "the medical profession has determined that death is a process rather than an event…physicians…conclude that patients reach a stage in the process of dying beyond which no chance of recovery exists. The cessation of total brain function known as brain death is widely accepted as constituting an irreversible stage in the process of dying."[44]

This view is accepted by Orthodox Jewish scholars who reason that just as decapitated animals may be viewed as dead even if "their limbs still jerk," so brain death may be viewed as physiological decapitation and therefore as indicating the death of the patient.[45] That being the case, keeping the patient on the respirator is merely ventilating a corpse. One should have no compunctions about removing such a patient from the ventilator.

Patients in an irreversible vegetative state present a somewhat different case because they are not clinically dead. If they have left no instructions about their end-of-life care, there is no way of knowing their intentions. If one believes that only the patient can decide about such matters, then one has no right to remove the patient from the respirator, thereby terminating both care and the patient.

The case of the fully conscious patient suffering from a "debilitating, progressive, and incurable disease" falls into the same category as the patient with Huntington's disease, and the same pattern of reasoning applies. If suicide is viewed as an acceptable option for that patient, it should be acceptable for this patient. The problem for the patient, however, is that of assistance. A patient in the early stage of Huntington's disease might amass sufficient drugs to commit suicide, but patient in a later stage would need someone else to procure them. Who that person will be may create a problem. Earlier we suggested that the physician be that person. Here, with the patient connected to a respirator, neither a relative nor a friend would be in a position to disconnect the patient. Therefore, it would be up to the physician to so act.

A final word: As anyone who has looked at the literature generated by this topic can attest, the arguments on this issue derive from a paucity of traditional texts that can be interpreted in more than one way. It is assumed that the texts describe real events and that conclusions derived from them are germane to our present situation. They may not be. The example of the *goses* is symbolic; how can a person expected to die within three days be instructive to the situation of the end-of-life patient who may linger in pain for weeks, if not months? In sum, if the technologies are different, how can lessons learned from one be applied to the other?

We have already seen that the supposed lessons are presented as "some" statements which do not have universal applicability. Therefore, the judging of any given problem has to be a matter of a cost-benefit analysis, just as in judging any other problem. Each situation must be judged on its own, assuming that we wish to maximize life where possible and avoid pain where possible. Where pain trumps life, where suffering cannot be controlled and recovery cannot be achieved, then if the patient feels that life is no longer worth living, and "the game not worth the candle," there is no need to extend life, and indeed, there may be a need to shorten it.

That decision is one which should be faced looking at the situation as it is in each particular case; some of the texts of the Jewish tradition may be useful and some may not. There is one text already quoted, that certainly may be useful: it is Rashi's understanding of the term "nice death"; in his view it meant that the afflicted person should *she-yamut maher*, "die quicker."[46]

Notes

1. Shimon Glick, "The Jewish Approach to Living and Dying," in *Jewish and Catholic Bio-Ethics: An Ecumenical Dialogue*, ed. E.D. Pellegrino and A.I. Faden (Washington, D.C.: Georgetown University Press, 1989), p. 43.

2. According to Rabbi Dr. Immanuel Jakobovits, "Jewish Attitudes to the Dying Patient," in *The European Colloquium in Medical Ethics: Jewish Perspectives*, ed. Avraham Steinberg (Jerusalem, Magnes Press. 1989), p. 42, "'Sanctity of life'...is a non-Jewish expression." On the other hand, Rabbi Dr. J. David Bleich, quoted by Ronald M. Green in "Jewish Teaching on the Sanctity and Quality of Life," in *Jewish and Catholic Bio-Ethics: An Ecumenical Dialogue*, ed. E.D. Pellegrino and A.I. Faden (Washington, D.C.: Georgetown University Press, 1989), p. 27, says that "Judaism teaches that human life is sacred from the moment of generation of genoplasm in the gonads until the decomposition after death."

3. Dr. Jakobovits holds that "euthanasia...is...plain murder." Immanuel Jakobovits, *Jewish Medical Ethics* (New York: Bloch Publishing Co., 1959), p. 123. Dr. Fred Rosner states that however laudable the intention of the person performing it, euthanasia is "an act of homicide." Fred Rosner, *Modern Medicine and Jewish Ethics* (Hoboken, NJ: Ktav, 1991), pp. 211–212.

4. E.g., Genesis 14:1, Numbers 31:6. Deuteronomy 20:2–4, Joshua 6:1, 10:12; Judges 5:9, I Samuel 4:6, II Samuel. 3:5.

5. Cf Mishnah Sotah 8:5. In his discussion of the kinds of war, in *Mishneh Torah*, Sefer Shoftim, Hilkhot Melakhim 5, Maimonides states that a king *may* engage in a *milhemet reshut*, a voluntary war, not only to extend the borders of the Land, but also to increase his own personal fame.

6. E.g., Leviticus 20:1 and 24:23.

7. Mishnah Sanhedrin 6–7.

8. *The Standard Jewish Encyclopedia*, ed. Cecil Roth (Garden City: NY: Doubleday, 1959), p. 403.

9. *The Standard Dictionary of the English Language, International Edition* (New York: Funk & Wagnalls Co., 1962), p. 836.

10. BT Sanhedrin 45a.

11. Leviticus 19:25. That an alternative to the death penalty might be an alternative approach to loving one's neighbor did not occur to the sages or the generations of readers of the talmudic passage.

12. BT Sanhedrin 45°, Rashi ad loc.

13. Israel Bettan, "Euthanasia," in *American Reform Responsa*, ed. Walter Jacob (New York: Central Conference of American Rabbis, 1983), pp. 261, 263. One of the discussants of Dr. Bettan's paper, Dr Samuel Atlas, argued that euthanasia was proscribed because creativity

was the distinguishing mark of human life and repentance was an act of creativity, and therefore "it is wrong to deprive a hopelessly sick person of the opportunity for repentance" (p. 267). The logic of Dr Atlas's position would be to refrain from providing any anodyne to "the hopelessly sick person" so as to make sure that person would be fully conscious to demonstrate creativity by properly repenting.

14. Rosner, *Modern Medicine and Jewish Ethics*, pp. 211–212. Note that "homicide" and "murder" have different meanings. For views similar to Rosner's, cf. S. Abraham, *The Comprehensive Guide to Medical Halakhah* (Jerusalem and New York, l990), p. 177; J. David Bleich, *Judaism and Healing: Halakhic Perspectives* (New York, 1981), pp. 135–136; Jakobovits, *Jewish Medical Ethics*, p. 123.

15. Mishnah Shabbat 23:5.

16. BT Shabbat 151b.

17. E.g., Bettan, "Euthanasia," p. 262; Rosner, *Modern Medicine and Jewish Ethics*, p. 206; Vishlitzky, L. *Madrikh Refui L'fee ha-Masoret ha-Yehudit* (Jerusalem, 1977), p. 87

18. Following the dating of H.L. Strack, *Introduction to Talmud and Midrash* (New York: Harper & Row, 1965), p. 113, Hananiah was martyred soon after the death of Akiba, i.e., about 135 C.E.; Judah the Prince lived from 135 to 193 C.E. (according to others, Judah died in 218 C.E. (p. 118); the name Yose (Ha-Galili) ben Halafta seems to be a conflate reading; there were a number of tannaim whose first name was Yose; if the intended person was Yose Ha-Galili, then his dates were somewhere from 90 to 130 C.E.; if the intended person was Yose ben Halafta, his dates were somewhere from 130 to 160 C.E. (pp. 113, 115).

19. BT Avodah Zarah 18b (author's translation). Rabbi Judah the Prince will be involved in another case of euthanasia below.

20. E.g., Bettan, "Euthanasia," p. 262; Rosner, *Modern Medicine and Jewish Ethics*, p. 206; Vishlitzky, *Madrikh Refui L'fee ha-Masoret ha-Yehudit*, p. 87.

21. Tosafot ad loc. suggests an exception to this teaching: if one feared that idolaters might use unbearable tortures to force a person to commit transgressions, it would then be licit, indeed a mitzvah (duty), to harm oneself. He gives the example (BT Gittin 57b) of the children, boys and girls, who to avoid being taken to Rome for a life of "shame" threw themselves into the sea. This exception has a number of interesting elements: The individuals involved fear that they will not be able to withstand something they are not suffering *at present* but which may occur in the future. The boys and girls in this tragic story had not at the moment of their death suffered torture or experienced the degradation of a life of shame; they ended their lives because of what they *anticipated*. One might deduce from this story that anticipated suffering is reason enough for suicide. Such a conclusion, to say the least, has not been drawn.

22. That the story of Hananiah has two conflicting elements was noted by David Gordis in "The Ethical in Jewish Bio-Ethics," *Judaism* 38, no. 1 (1989): 28–40. Dr. Gordis also saw the contractual nature of the discussion with the executioner and related the discussion to the supposed difference between active and passive euthanasia. Dr. Israel Bettan, "Euthanasia," p. 265, saw the conflicting elements of the story as such a difference. Dr. Gordis, however, noted that "'The most obvious objection to reading this narrative (T.B. Avodah Zarah 18a) as a rabbinic endorsement of distinguishing between active and passive euthanasia is the reported behavior of Rabbi Hananiah himself. After all, is it so clear that his merely opening his mouth constitutes something along the lines of active euthanasia, while the contract with the executioner is passive?"

23. BT Ketubbot 104a. Rashi, ad loc., explains that Rabbi was suffering from an intestinal complaint.
24. About Rabbi's maid, Dr. Rosner wrote, "This woman is reported to have prayed for his death," *Jewish Bio-Ethics*, 1979, p. 271. He omits the fact that she "is reported" to have acted! Dr. Bleich wrote that the maid "is depicted in rabbinic writings as a woman of exemplary piety and moral character. This woman is reported to have prayed for his death" (*Judaism and Healing*, p. 142). He also does not mention that she did more than pray, she acted. He did note that after she "expressed her feelings and conveyed information about her master's pain and discomfort to his disciples, they not only declined to join her in prayer for his decease, but did not desist in praying for the prolongation of his life" (ibid., p. 143). It is instructive to note what Drs. Rosner and Bleich extract and fail to extract from the passage; indeed, Dr. Bleich's grasp of detail is significant for what it omits.
25. The Talmud text does not contain what h we find in another text, viz. "Jewish Law... cannot...purchase relief from pain and misery at the cost of life itself." Jakobovitz, *Jewish Medical Ethics*, p. 275. The story of Rabbi's death is precisely about "relief from pain and misery at the cost of life itself."
26. *Yalkut Shimoni*, with introduction by Bezalel Landoy (Jerusalem, 1960), vol. 2, sec. 943, p. 980. The passage continues, "Therefore, Solomon said, 'Happy is the man who hearkens to me' (Ps. 8:34) [the point is found in the continuation of the verse, 'Watching daily at my gates, waiting at the post of my doors.'] What is written after that? 'He who finds Me, finds life' (Ps. 8:35)." The continuation of the first verse and the second verse quoted suggest that attendance at the synagogue is a means of preserving life. If so, not going to the synagogue would be a way of ending life.
27. BT Gittin 28a. The legal consequences in this passage relate to the assumption that a husband who was a *goses* was alive when a bill of divorce was delivered. The presumption of mortality of the *goses* is quoted as a factor in oath taking in BT Shevuot 37b. Rashi, ad loc., states that the *goses* while not dead is to be treated as if alive in every matter.
28. Semahot, chap. 1. This translation is taken from *The Minor Tractates of the Talmud* (London: Soncino Press, 1965), vol. 1, pp. 326–327. According to a later authority, Joshua Falk, quoted in Jakobovitz, *Jewish Medical Ethics*, p. 121 (in text) and (in notes) p. 349, n. 18, the period of being a *goses* is but three days.
29. Isserles, gloss on the *Shulhan Arukh*, Yoreh Deah 339, as quoted in Rosner, *Modern Medicine and Jewish Ethics*, p. 207.
30. Rosner, *Modern Medicine and Jewish Ethics*, p. 198, writes, "Passive euthanasia is defined as the situation in which therapy is withheld so that death is hastened by omission of treatment." However, in the examples cited by Isserles of the removal of the impediments to death, there is no "omission of treatment." Rosner also notes (p. 208) that "the discontinuation of life-support systems which are specifically designed and utilized in the treatment of incurably ill patients might only be permissible if one is certain that in doing so one is shortening the act of dying and not interrupting life." The distinction between "the act of dying" and "life" seems to be the difference between the three-day or seventy-hour life expectancy of the *goses* and the more extended life of a patient. Even so, perhaps because he is a practicing physician, Rosner seems to suggest more flexibility than other writers. One is reminded of a line in a speech given in a euthanasia debate in the House of Lords, "The good doctor is aware of the difference between prolonging

life and prolonging the act of dying," quoted in Glanville Williams, *The Sanctity of Life and the Criminal Law* (New York, 1968), pp. 336–337.

31. Cf. above, n. 28.

32. Glick, *Jewish Approach to Living and Dying*, p. 36, contrasts past end-of-life decisions with present end-of-life decisions saying, "We both know the fatal outcome with certainty and can forestall it indefinitely."

33. Rosner, *Modern Medicine and Jewish Ethics*, p. 210.

34. Thus, Dr. Bleich deduces from the case of the guilty *sotah* who suffered in a "debilitating and degenerative state, which led to a protracted termination of life," that "life accompanied by pain is thus viewed as preferable to death." Bleich, *Judaism and Healing*, pp. 135–136

35. *Tzitz Eliezer*, IX, no 47, sec. 5, quoted in Bleich, *Judaism and Healing*, p. 137, and Rosner, *Modern Medicine and Jewish Ethics*, pp. 210–211

36. Leon R. Kass, "Death with Dignity and the Sanctity of Life," in *A Time to Be Born and a Time to Die: The Ethics of Choice*, ed. Barry S. Kogan (New York: Aldine de Gruyter, 1991), p. 128.

37. Glick, *Jewish Approach to Living and Dying*, p. 46.

38. Judges 16:30.

39. I Samuel 31:4–5.

40. BT Gittin 57b. Cf. n. 21 above.

41. Psalm 44:23.

42. Walter Jacob, "Huntington's Disease and Suicide," in *Death and Euthanasia in Jewish Law*, ed. Walter Walter and Moshe Zemer (Pittsburgh and Tel Aviv: Freehof Institute of Progressive Halacha, Rodef Shalom Press, 1995), p. 135. Also, Walter Jacob, *Contemporary Reform Responsa* (New York, 1981), no. 81.

43. Webster's *Ninth New Collegiate Dictionary* (Springfield, Mass.: Merriam-Webster, 1983), p. 1180.

44. P.L. Ryan, "The Uniform Determination of Death Act: An Effective Solution to the Problem of Defining Death," *Washington & Lee Law Review* 39 (1982): 1512, quoted in Moshe Zemer, "Determining Death in Jewish Law," in *Death and Euthanasia*, ed. Walter Jacob and Moshe Zemer (Pittsburgh and Tel Aviv: Rodef Shalom Press, 1995), p. 110, n. 15, p. 119.

45. Moshe Tendler, quoting Mishnah Ohalot 1:6 in *Death and Euthanasia*, ed. Walter Jacob and Moshe Zemer (Pittsburgh and Tel Aviv: Rodef Shalom Press, 1995), p. 111 and in the notes, p. 119; idem, "Cessation of Brain Function: Ethical Implications in Terminal Care and Organ Transplant," *Annals of the New York Academy of Sciences* (New York, 1978), pp. 394–395. Similarly, the *Journal of the American Medical Association* 240 (1977): 1651 explains that the complete and irreversible destruction of the brain, which includes the loss of all its function, can be considered physiological decapitation and thus a determinant *per se* of death.

46. Above, n. 10.

A Law Proposal in Israel Regarding the Patient at the End of Life

THE STEINBERG COMMITTEE

Avraham Steinberg

T HE MORAL, halakhic, sociocultural, and legal aspects of the treatment of the dying patient are among the most difficult and widely discussed topics in modern medicine, encompassing tens of books, hundreds of declarations, directives, laws, and judgments, and thousands of professional and nonprofessional articles in the realms of medicine, philosophy, law, sociology, and religion.

Although the approach to the dying patient has been one of the most prominent problems in medicine since time immemorial, the dilemma has been intensified in the past few decades. This is due to the enormous advances in medicine and technology, the transformation of the patient-physician relationship from paternalistic to autonomous, the massive involvement of various professionals in the treatment of the dying patient, and the many economic and cultural changes in recent years.

On February 20, 2000, the minister of health, Shlomo Benizri, appointed Prof. Avraham Steinberg to head a national committee charged with formulating a law that would regulate all matters concerning the dying patient in Israel. The trigger for the establishment of this committee was the case of Itai Arad, an Israeli pilot suffering from amyotrophic lateral sclerosis (ALS), who was intubated and asked for the respirator to be withdrawn. A local ethics committee turned down the request, but Judge Moshe Talgam of the Tel Aviv district court approved it. For the first time in Israel a respirator was withdrawn from a respirator-dependent patient in an overt and open manner. The patient died within several hours. A heated debate followed in the Knesset (Israeli parliament) and in the media.

During the several years before this event about twenty cases involving dying patients were discussed and settled by court decisions. These, however, were individual decisions with no constitutional basis. Several attempts were made to settle issues related to the dying patient by law, but they all failed for various reasons.

Thus, the establishment of the committee created great expectations among law-makers and the public at large.

Following is a brief summary of the committee's organizational structure and functions, and of the main points of the law it proposed:

The committee had fifty-nine members, making it the largest committee ever established in Israel for a specific issue. Every member of the committee was an expert, a ranking professional in some relevant field. All the relevant disciplines were represented. The members represented the entire spectrum of relevant views in Israel. None of them was a political or otherwise interested appointee. For close to two years (April 2000 to January 2002) intense debates took place. Every opinion and viewpoint was freely expressed and seriously discussed with great mutual respect. The debates and discussions were all closed to the media, and moreover, there were no leaks to the media during the entire process of formulating the proposed law. This was an important factor in enabling totally free communication and expression of opinions. There was a serious attempt by all members to reach as wide a consensus as possible despite the very difficult and emotionally-laden issues at stake.

The committee membership included forty-five men and fourteen women. Fifty-six were Jewish, one Christian, one Muslim, and one Druse. Of the Jewish members, thirty-four were secular, seventeen were Orthodox, three were ultra-Orthodox, one Conservative, and one Reform.

The chairman of the committee was Prof. Avraham Steinberg, pediatric neurologist at the Shaare Zedek Medical Center, Jerusalem, medical ethicist at Hebrew University-Hadassah Medical School, Jerusalem, and Israel Prize laureate.[1]

The committee was divided into four subcommittees:

The medical/scientific subcommittee, headed by Prof. Charles Sprung, M.D., director of the Intensive Care Unit at Hadassah Medical Center, Jerusalem, and chairman of ethics at the European Society of Intensive Care Medicine. The twenty-six members of were physicians, nurses, social workers, and sociologists. The physicians represented every field of medicine that deals with dying patients (intensive care, palliative medicine, cardiology, geriatrics, anesthesiology, psychiatry, pediatrics, neonatology, rehabilitation, oncology, neurology, and hospital management).

The philosophical/ethical subcommittee was headed by Prof. Asa Kasher, head of ethics in the Philosophy Department at Tel Aviv University and Israel Prize laureate. The twelve members were philosophers, medical ethicists, and clergy from different religions (Jewish Reform and Conservative, Christian Greek Orthodox, Islam, and Druse).

The legal subcommittee was headed by Prof. Amnon Carmi, former district court judge in Haifa, president of the Israeli Society of Medicine and Law, and chair of the International Center for Health Law and Ethics. The thirteen members were judges, lawyers, professors of law, and legal advisers of relevant ministries.

The halakhic (Jewish law) subcommittee was headed by Rabbi Yaacov Ariel, chief rabbi of Ramat-Gan. The seven members were rabbis and physicians well versed in matters of medicine and halakhah.

The members of each subcommittee discussed all relevant matters from their specific professional standpoints. The subcommittees held thirty-five meetings. Over twenty scientific papers were submitted by members in order to better explain relevant facts and positions.

The entire committee convened three times to discuss the proposed law. There were six full drafts before the final version of the proposed law was presented to the minister of health, Nissim Dahan, on January 17, 2002.

The proposed law contains over a hundred paragraphs. It is a comprehensive document setting forth principles and practical applications that represent an appropriate balance between opposing values and positions. Despite the inherent complexity of the subject from the medical, moral, philosophical, religious, legal, sociocultural, and psychological standpoints, and despite the deep differences of opinion between members of the committee deriving from their diverse backgrounds and philosophical/ethical positions, we managed to reach a wide consensus on most issues related to the proposed law. Eighty percent of the members agreed on all the paragraphs of the proposed law; and all of the members agreed on 95 percent of the paragraphs. The only significant dissenting opinion pertained to the issue of withdrawing continuous treatment from a dying patient. Although in principle there is still a disagreement on this issue, with a minority opinion accepting the principle that there is no difference between withholding and withdrawing any therapy, we managed to minimize the practical disagreement by accepting the idea of a timer attached to a respirator.[2]

Thus it gives great satisfaction to note that the committee was successful in reaching a wide consensus on the most difficult issue in medical ethics. This was so because the members engaged in a serious debate in which views were expressed openly with no publicity during the discussions. The outcome demonstrates the good intentions and strong determination of all members of the committee to reach a workable and balanced solution to a very difficult issue.

The basic assumption of the proposed law is that most people do not want to die, but similarly that most people do not want to suffer at the end of life, and do not want their lives to be prolonged artificially without purpose.

From a philosophical/moral point of view, it is necessary to find an appropriate balance between opposing values and principles on such matters as the sanctity of life, the quality of life, autonomy, beneficence, nonmaleficence, distributive justice, and the slippery slope. The proposed law sanctions life by prohibiting any action that intentionally shortens it, such as active euthanasia, physician-assisted suicide, or the withdrawal of a continuous treatment such as a pacemaker or a respirator. On the other hand, the proposed law enables an autonomous decision to withhold any treatment directly related to the dying process, including the withholding of intermittent treatments, such as dialysis or chemotherapy, even after they are initiated. The proposed law requires palliative treatment even if it might sometimes unintentionally shorten life.

From a Jewish-religious point of view, it is necessary to determine the boundaries of responsibility for prolonging life versus the avoidance of unjustifiable suffering. The proposed law is based upon the rulings of three of the most authoritative decisors (*posekim*) of our generation, Rabbi Moshe Feinstein, Rabbi Shlomo Zalman Auerbach, and Rabbi Shmuel Wasner. According to relevant halakhic principles and the actual rulings of these very prominent rabbis, preserving life is one of the most important values, but it is not an infinitive or an absolute value. Any act that shortens life is halakhically considered to be murder, even at the very end of life (*goses*). Therefore, active euthanasia, physician-assisted suicide, or the withdrawal of a continuous treatment such as a pacemaker or a respirator is absolutely forbidden. On the other hand, there is no obligation to actively prolong the pain and suffering of a dying patient. Thus, it is permissible to withhold any treatment directly related to the dying process, including the intermittent treatments, such as dialysis or chemotherapy, even after they have been initiated.

From a medical-scientific point of view, it is necessary to define various medical situations and treatments as well as to execute legal directions and decisions. Therefore, the proposed law requires the appointment of a senior physician as the responsible person to analyze all the relevant facts, in cooperation with relevant experts and decision-makers, so to formulate a detailed plan of commission and omission, and to document these decisions in a clear and overt manner.

From a social-cultural point of view, it is necessary to resolve issues concerning competent and incompetent patients in relation to decision-makers, and to establish problem-solving mechanisms for a variety of situations. Therefore, the proposed law establishes a hierarchy of decision-making. In the case of competent dying patients, the patient's wishes take precedence over any other mode of decision-making; in the case of incompetent dying patients, decisions should be based on advance medical directives or a surrogate appointed by the patient while competent. Testimony about the incompetent dying patient's wishes by family members or friends known to be close to the patient is also acceptable. Local and national ethics committees are the proposed problem-solving mechanism.

It is beyond the scope of this introductory summary to deal with the proposed law in detail. Suffice it to say that the proposed law contains definitions, determinations, and solutions to all the above-mentioned issues and to many others as well, and provides innovative solutions to the difficult problems posed by dying patients.

On March 21, 2004 the law proposed by the committee was accepted by the Israeli government and became the official governmental proposal of the Act Concerning the Dying Patient, 2004. It is now up to the Knesset to enact this proposal as law in Israel, modify it, or reject it.

It is my hope that the law will be enacted as proposed by the committee without significant and fundamental changes, because it represents the best balance between the opposing views in Israel and offers adequate and acceptable solutions to almost every issue concerning the dying patient.

The Law Proposal of the Steinberg Committee together with its history, main discussions, and divergent opinions appears in the appendix.

Notes

1. The highest and most prestigious price for scientific, cultural, or social achievement in Israel
2. Vardit Ravitsky's essay "Dying with Dignity in a Jewish-Democratic State" in this book deals extensively with this point

Dying with Dignity in a Jewish-Democratic State

Vardit Ravitsky

Introduction

Modern medicine is one of the greatest successes of the past century. It has eradicated a few life-threatening diseases, almost doubled the average life expectancy in many developed countries, and can, to date, effectively treat numerous conditions. As a result, we have learned to trust it and rely on it. Moreover, most of us will put ourselves in the hands of health-care providers at one of the most vulnerable times of our lives – the time of our death. While performing wonders for us during our lives, modern medicine has the power to harshly intervene in the painful and intimate process of dying. It can prolong suffering and sometimes makes it difficult to preserve human dignity in face of the inevitable.

During the weeks in which my grandfather of blessed memory lay unconscious connected to a ventilator in an intensive care unit following head surgery, I would stand at his bedside and feel tortured at the sight of his suffering. The loving grandpa who had always been there for me, the respectable-looking man in the elegant suit, was gone. Only his body lay there in agony, the ventilator pumping air into his lungs. At the sight of his chest going up and down in a rhythm dictated by the ventilator, and the sight of his unspoken discomfort and anguish, I asked myself whether this was the way he would have chosen to end his life. Dignity was of paramount importance to him throughout his life. Was this the last memory he would have wanted to leave behind for his children and grandchildren?

End-of-life care and the right to die with dignity have become two of the most controversial issues in bioethics in recent years. While many questions about biomedical technology seem to be futuristic or esoteric, end-of-life questions touch on the lives of everyone. Many people find themselves struggling with these questions while going through the painful process of taking farewell from a loved one, as in the case of my beloved grandfather, years before they are confronted with their own death.

Consequently, end-of-life questions tend to fuel an intense public debate in many countries. Public attitudes are usually based on cultural narratives and moral values (often stemming from a religious background) that nourish the social texture. I would like to argue that any attempt to legislate or regulate issues of moral and social weight should be attuned to the cultural, moral, and religious circumstances in which it occurs. Policy-makers in a democratic state should take into consideration not only professional expert opinions, but also the social and cultural context in which they are operating.

To date, end-of-life care is not regulated by legislation in Israel. In light of the lack of a coherent policy and the growing concern, Israel's health minister established a public committee in 2000 to formulate guidelines for end-of-life care.[1] In 2002, the Public Committee Regarding the Patient at the End of Life submitted its recommendations in the form of a law proposal. This paper will demonstrate how the proposed law expresses sensitivity to the cultural circumstances in which it was created, and will analyze the ethical and philosophical meaning of one compromise that it proposes. The focus of the discussion will be on the highly controversial issue of withdrawing care versus withholding it.

The Israeli Social Reality

In its Basic Law: Human Dignity and Freedom, Israel defines itself as a "Jewish democratic state." One meaning of this proclamation is that in the development of public policy and legislation, particularly with regard to issues that have profound moral and social implications, the state is supposed to seek a synthesis of Jewish and democratic values. In the case of end-of-life care, this requires weighing the value of personal autonomy and the right of individuals to determine what care they will receive or refuse to receive, against the religious conception of the infinite value of human life, or "sanctity of life."

In the end-of-life context, both sets of values have far-reaching implications. The value of autonomy has special weight when we make the ultimate decision about how and when to end our life, and when our dignity is at stake. On the other hand, the religious conception of life as given to human beings by God and therefore as "belonging" to God, has very different implications for what we can and cannot choose to do at the end of our life. The biblical imperative of "therefore choose life"[1] may be perceived in this context as obliging us not to take any action to shorten the process of dying. Although these two conceptual frameworks may seem to be incompatible, the Public Committee Regarding the Patient at the End of Life sought a way of striking a balance that everyone can live with.

Another important factor in understanding the fabric of Israeli society is its communitarian tendency, which sometimes leads toward a certain degree of social paternalism. As Gross notes:

> To this day in Israel, collectivism remains an overriding norm.... Although Israel's paternalism is not heavy-handed...collective concerns are nevertheless often admitted to override individual interests.... Communitarian dialogue pushes...to *alter* the individual's preferences to better harmonize with the collective voice – not necessarily to advance the collective interest, but to reflect the collective assessment of what is best for the individual.[2]

This tendency is strongly reflected in the Patients Rights Act of 1996,[3] in which informed consent for medical treatment is deemed necessary, while at the same time the law permits an ethics committee to override the wishes of a competent adult patient not to be treated, in the name of a social understanding of the patient's "best interests."[4]

Israeli Legal Reality and the Proposed Law

As noted earlier, end-of-life care is currently not regulated by legislation in Israel. The Patients Rights Act of 1996 excludes any mention of patients' rights at the end of life, and criminal law forbids any action that accelerates a patient's death.

When examining the Israeli legal approach, one should distinguish between cases that involve active euthanasia (i.e., any measure aimed at actively hastening death) or any form of assisted suicide, and cases that involve passive euthanasia (i.e., withholding or withdrawing treatment at the end of life). To date, the Israeli legal system clearly objects to any type of active euthanasia and assisted suicide. It considers such acts to be forms of killing or murder. However, with regard to the withholding and withdrawing of treatment, the approach of the courts has not always been consistent.

In general, Israeli courts have been reluctant to affirm requests relating to minors. In some cases, the courts have affirmed the request of a competent, terminally ill patient to refuse ventilator support on grounds that the treatment is extraordinary, heroic, and probably futile. Moreover, in other cases, the courts have permitted the *removal* of life support from once-competent patients who were careful to document their intentions well before losing consciousness.[5]

As noted above, in light of the lack of a coherent policy, a multidisciplinary public committee was established to formulate guidelines for the care of terminally ill patients with a remaining life span of six months or less. Despite the dissenting opinions, the committee sought consensus and a delicate balance between Jewish and democratic values. In the introductory remarks to the proposal, Professor Steinberg, the committee's chair, writes:

> The committee's assumption is that from a social and a national point of view, it is appropriate to reach solutions for the problem of end-of-life care, based on a wide consensus, while balancing the conflicting values which underlie decision-making processes in this area. In the State of Israel there is a unique need to reach agreement based on its value system as a Jewish democratic state.[6]

The result of the committee's work is a long and complex document, proposing detailed legislation that will regulate many aspects of end-of-life care. The proposed law addresses such issues as competent and incompetent patients, advanced directive and durable power of attorney, the role of family and friends in end-of-life decision-making, the role of ethics committees, and the need for appropriate palliative care.[7]

This paper will focus on one aspect of the proposed law: the distinction between continuous and discrete care as a basis for the distinction between withholding and withdrawing treatment.

Continuous vs. Discrete Care

The proposed law distinguishes "continuous care," defined as any form of care that is essentially uninterrupted and admits of no clear distinction between the end of one cycle and the beginning of another, and "discrete care," defined as care that does begin and end in well-defined cycles. The prime example of continuous care is mechanical ventilation.

This distinction is of paramount importance to the law, since it delineates limits imposed upon an autonomous competent adult patient who makes end-of-life decisions. According to the proposed law, such a patient is permitted to refuse discrete care (i.e., to request the withholding of care), but not to request the termination or cessation of continuous care (i.e., the withdrawing of care). Being disconnected from a ventilator is therefore a choice that the law does not allow. Section 12 says: "It is forbidden to terminate continuous medical care (unless it is done for the purpose of medical treatment), when the termination may lead to the death of the patient, whether competent or not competent; however, it is permitted to terminate discrete care, under the conditions set in section 13."[8]

A legal reality in which a competent adult patient who has been connected to a ventilator (whether at the patient's own request or against patient's will) cannot be disconnected, is extremely problematic for at least two reasons. First, on the level of principle, the proposed law does not respect an important aspect of personal autonomy at a crucial time of life. Second, on a practical level, it may lead to situations in which patients refuse to be connected to a ventilator in the first place, from fear that once connected they will be trapped in an endless cycle of suffering against their will.

This very dilemma occurred when my grandfather was lying unconscious in an intensive care unit. One morning my phone rang and I heard my grandmother crying. A nurse had just explained to her that my grandfather's breathing was deteriorating fast and a decision had to be made about whether to connect him to a ventilator. No other family member was present at the time, and the decision had to be made immediately. The physician at the other end of the line made it clear to me that "once connected, we will not be able to disconnect."

This personal story exemplifies the dilemma many families face. In the Israeli normative reality, the message is clear: you may choose not to be connected, but once connected your circumstances are irreversible. This leads to situations in which a decision of such magnitude is made in haste, without appropriate discussion among family members. Moreover, in case of doubt it may lead to a decision not to connect, because the patient or family members would rather avoid the possibility of prolonged suffering and loss of dignity than gain a few more hours, days, or weeks of life.

This is not only true for patients and their families, but may also be relevant to health-care providers. As the British Medical Association points out: "There is a risk that the perceived difficulty of withdrawing treatment could lead to some patients failing to receive treatment which could benefit them.... some health professionals may be reluctant to start treatment in the mistaken belief that, once initiated, the treatment cannot be withdrawn."[9]

This point was made by a few dissenting members of the public committee Regarding the Patient at the End of Life in their comments on the proposed law. For example, Judge Talgam asked that the following section be added to the proposal:

"It is permitted to withdraw treatment if the patient is competent and requests the withdrawal, or if the treatment was given without the patient's explicit consent and the patient is now competent and changes his mind, or it is clear that the patient did not want the treatment in the first place."[10]

Prof. Avinoam Rekhes recommended "dispens[ing] with the distinction between continuous and discrete care and...allow[ing] disconnection from a ventilator under appropriate sedation," claiming that otherwise "there will be no appropriate solution for an ALS [define] [Amyotrophic Lateral Sclerosis, a rapidly progressive paralyes leading to death] patient who wants to end his life in full competence and awareness."[11]

Dr. Carmel Shalev made a similar request to dispense with the distinction, emphasizing that "Just as informed consent is required before giving medical care, and just as care should not be given against a patient's will, it is also forbidden to coerce patients into continuing treatment when it is obvious that they do not want it. In both cases, enforcing treatment is a violation of the right to bodily integrity and constitutes assault according to existing law."[12]

Prof. Amos Shapira concurred and added an idea for a practical solution: "to allow medical institutions that operate based on the principles of religious tradition, and have an explicit and publicly declared policy that opposes withdrawal of care, to act in such a manner with regard to their hospitalized patients."[13] The underlying idea is, of course, to establish transparency in order to allow patients the choice of an appropriate hospital according to their own values and beliefs.

The question of continuous care and the prohibition of withdrawal thus generated numerous dissenting opinions by committee members who felt that this aspect of the proposed law poses a real threat to personal autonomy and to patient's rights. As Judge Talgam points out:

> There is no doubt that the establishment of the committee and the formulation of its findings constitute efforts to "live together."...
> However, the dichotomic picture presented by chairman – as if we are speaking of a spectrum on which each party should make some concessions and then all will be well – is too optimistic. The work of the committee defined the area in which it is *possible* to

reach agreement – it left the rest as separate worlds in which each party has its own *red lines*.[14]

Western Bioethics vs. the Israeli Attitude

Key features of this Israeli debate depart from currently well accepted bioethical norms in most Western countries. Whereas in Israeli culture (as is apparent in the proposed law) the distinction between continuous and discrete care (or withholding and withdrawing care) remains important, in most cases Western bioethical literature no longer acknowledges this distinction.

As early as 1983, an American court acknowledged the right to withdraw treatment. The presiding judge argued that "each pulsation of the respirator or each drop of fluid introduced into the patient's body by intravenous feeding devices is comparable to a manually administered injection or item of medication."[15]

The judge's argument makes it possible to see that withdrawing treatment, a contentious idea at the time, is nothing more than refusing treatment, an already well founded moral and legal right. Since then, the distinction between refusing treatment and refusing to continue treatment has largely disappeared and no longer carries ethical and legal weight in most Western countries.

For example, in a document entitled "Withholding and Withdrawing Life Prolonging Medical Treatment: Guidance for Decision Making," published in 1999 by the British Medical Association, the distinction is explicitly rejected: "Although emotionally it may be easier to withhold treatment than to withdraw that which has been started, there are no legal, or necessary morally relevant, differences between the two actions…. In fact, withdrawal of life-prolonging treatment is often morally safer than withholding it."[16]

In Israel, however, for a variety of cultural, religious, and symbolic reasons, the distinction continues to play a central role. As Gross point out:

> In general the courts and medical practitioners continue to draw
> sharp distinctions between withholding and withdrawing treat-

ment.... They disapprove of withdrawing life support from any patient.... And while some district courts have recently sought to expand a patient's right to discontinue life support, these decisions were rejected outright by the Israel Medical Association in order to "preserve the moral integrity of physicians and prevent a slide down the slippery slope."[17]

Other countries acknowledge the emotional aspect of the distinction:

Although there may be no legal or moral difference between withholding and withdrawing treatment when making decisions about an individual patient, this is not to say that emotionally and psychologically the two are equivalent. Many health professionals, as well as patients, feel an emotional difference between withholding and withdrawing treatment. This is likely to be linked to the largely negative impression attached to a decision to withdraw treatment, which can be interpreted as abandonment or "giving up on the patient."[18]

The British guidelines acknowledge the tension between the emotional and the rational. An individual physician may accept the philosophical and legal arguments leading to the rejection of the distinction on moral grounds, but when faced with the prospect of having to disconnect an individual patient from a ventilator, may still face emotional and psychological difficulties.

The tension between moral reasoning and intuitive personal reactions requires some attention. The solution offered by Western bioethics is generally to overcome the emotional difficulty by educating oneself to emphasize the weight of rational reasoning. For example, the British Medical Association's guidelines suggest that "Greater emphasis on the reasons for providing treatment...and greater clarity about the legitimate scope and process of decision making by health professionals are likely to challenge this perceived difference."[19]

The Israeli reality is different in this respect. First, the Israeli social reality is one with strongly communitarian tendencies. Therefore, the value of individual personal autonomy does not carry enough cultural weight to encourage such an "educational move" within the medical community and within public opinion.

Second, the deeply ingrained roots of this distinction in Halakhah (Orthodox Jewish religious law) make it powerful in the context of Israeli culture, which aspires to embrace Jewish tradition and Jewish values into the democratic process of policy-aking. Thus, the proposed law takes a different approach to this tension.

Timers on Ventilators: Transforming the Continuous Into Discrete Treatment

Instead of attempting to educate the medical community and the public to disregard the distinction between continuous and discrete care, committee members looked to a mechanical technical solution. They came up with the idea of transforming the continuous into the discrete (in the case of ventilation) by installing timers on the machines.

Following this idea the Public Committee Regarding the Patient at the End of Life established the Committee for Transforming Ventilation into Discrete Medical Treatment. The goal of this new committee was defined as finding a mechanical solution that will lead to the installation of delayed-response timers on ventilators. The timers would make it possible to set the ventilator in advance for only a limited period of time, thus turning ventilation into a "discrete" type of care.

In one of the reports submitted by the committee, its chair, Dr. Halperin (the chief officer for medical ethics in the Ministry of Health), noted that "Not renewing treatment that has been interrupted, can be defined as withholding treatment."[20] The committee emphasized, however, that this mechanical solution should in no way endanger the lives of patients and should not allow unplanned interruptions of the ventilators to occur.

Once developed and installed, the timers will make Israel the first and only country in the world to implement a policy that offers a mechanical-technical solution to the cultural issues raised by the distinction between withholding and withdrawing ventilation. What is the ethical meaning of this solution? Are timers deceptive devices meant to disguise an immoral act as a legitimate one? Will they enable Israeli physicians to perform in practice what their moral intuitions forbid them from doing in principle?

As mentioned earlier, the Public Committee Regarding the Patient at the End of Life was nominated in order to find a solution that embraces both Jewish and democratic values. Even though the distinction between withholding and withdrawing care is no longer acknowledged as carrying any moral or legal weight in Western bioethics, I would argue that committee members were right to take into consideration the attitudes of the Israeli medical community and of significant elements of the Israeli public. As argued earlier, a democratic process of legislation and regulation should be sensitive to the cultural context in which it takes place.

Second, a philosophical analysis reveals that criticism of the timers as "deceptive" is justified only if we assign moral weight to the underlying distinction. If the distinction carries moral weight (in the sense that withdrawal of care is morally wrong, whereas withholding care is morally permitted), then a device that transforms what is, in essence, withdrawing into what only externally looks like withholding, has problematic ethical implications.

If the medical community's reluctance to disconnect a patient from a ventilator is based on the fact that disconnecting is indeed ethically wrong, then it is appropriate to perceive the timers as disguising the true nature of the act. On this assumption, timers will create an emotional distance from the "wrongness" of the act and will enable professionals to overcome their justified ethical inclination by using a ruse, thus eroding a well-founded moral intuition.

If the distinction carries moral weight, then the problem of disconnecting a patient from a ventilator should be confronted directly and the appropriate price should be paid in terms of limits to individual autonomy. In such a case, evading the real issue by creating a mechanical illusion that disguises A as B allows professionals to dodge their moral responsibility. In short, if the distinction is ethically significant, then timers will have a negative educational impact on the medical community, allowing providers to become emotionally accustomed to wrongdoing.

However, if the distinction is erroneous, as argued throughout the Western bioethical literature, then timers may be perceived as devices that enable individuals to overcome an emotional difficulty in order to do what is ethically right. They thus become an appropriate and clever way to bridge the gap between the desired moral outcome (death with dignity and respect for individual autonomy) and a cultural atmosphere (grounded in religious tradition and ingrained values) that does not allow renunciation of the distinction.

Conclusion

End-of-life care is a complex and socially sensitive issue that raises many ethical dilemmas. Israel's Public Committee Regarding the Patient at the End of Life was appointed in order to fill a regulatory vacuum, with the goal of drafting a law proposal, based on the widest possible consensus and reflecting a balance of Jewish and democratic values.

This paper explores one specific aspect of the committee's proposal: the attempt to respect the cultural distinction between withholding and withdrawing care, while finding a practical technical solution for patients who choose to be disconnected from a ventilator in order to end their lives with dignity. I argue that the mechanical solution of installing timers on ventilators is ethically appropriate and should not be criticized as either deceptive or morally corruptive.

A short analysis revealed that such criticisms are valid only if the distinction is assumed to carry moral weight. However, in current Western bioethics, valid moral arguments have led to a policy that does not acknowledge the distinction. In most Western countries today, withdrawing care is perceived as morally equivalent to withholding care. Both acts are considered to be respectful of the individual patient's autonomy.

A mechanical device that will allow the Israeli medical community to overcome the cultural and emotional barriers to doing what is ethically right, therefore, is an insightful and clever solution. It allows policy-makers to bridge the gap between the imperative of personal autonomy and the need to respect cultural and social values in the process of policy-making. Timers on ventilators constitute an appropriate novel solution that paves the way for the successful integration of Jewish and democratic values.

Notes

1. Of which I was a member.
2. L. Michael Gross, "Autonomy and Paternalism in Communitarian Society: Patient Rights in Israel," *Hastings Center Report* 29, no. 4 (1999): 17–18.
3. Israel Patients Rights Act, 1996. SH 5756, p. 327.
4. Section 15 of the Patients' Rights Act enables physicians to treat competent adult patients against their explicit wishes under the following circumstances: (1) the patient refuses treatment even though in "severe danger" (i.e., death or permanent disability), and (2) the ethics committee has heard the patient and determined that (a) the treatment is likely to significantly improve the patient's condition, (b) the patient has been given the information necessary for informed consent, (c) there are grounds to assume that the patient will "consent retroactively" (i.e., will express satisfaction after the fact regarding the treatment received against his/her initially expressed will).
5. *Bibas v. The Attorney General of Israel* (1997), HP 528/96, and *Idit Meir v. The Attorney General of Israel* (1998), HP 401/98.
6. Report of the Public Committee Regarding the Patient at the End of Life, p. 7. The full proposal is given in the appendix of this book.
7. *Proposed Law: The Patient at the End of Life* (Jerusalem: Public Committee for Issues Related to Patients at the End of Life, 2002), pars. 12–13.
8. Section 13 says: "It is permitted to withhold medical care that is related to the untreatable condition of the end-of-life patient...including resuscitation, connection to a ventilator, chemotherapy and radiation, dialysis, surgery. etc." The same section forbids, however, withholding care that is not related to the untreatable medical condition and also forbids withholding nutrition and hydration in any form.
9. British Medical Association, *Withholding and Withdrawing Life Prolonging Medical Treatment: Guidance for Decision Making*, 2nd ed. (London: BMJ Books, 2001), pp.: 12–14.
10. Report of the Public Committee Regarding the Patient at the End of Life, dissenting opinions, Judge Moshe Talgam, p. 18.
11. Ibid., dissenting opinions, Prof. Avinoam Rekhes, p. 19.
12. Ibid., dissenting opinions, Dr. Carmel Shalev, p. 20.
13. Ibid., dissenting opinions, Prof. Amos Shapira, p. 21.
14. Moshe Talgam, "Proposed Law on End of Life: Bridge or Coercion?" *Medicine and Law* 28 (2003): 39 (in Hebrew).
15. *Barber v. The Superior Court of Los Angeles County*, 147 Cal. App 3d 1006 (1983).
16. British Medical Association. *Withholding and Withdrawing Life Prolonging Medical Treatment*, pp. 12–14.

17. Gross, "Autonomy and Paternalism in Communitarian Society," p. 15.

18. British Medical Association, *Withholding and Withdrawing Life Prolonging Medical Treatment*, pp. 12–14.

19. Ibid.

20. Mordechai Halperin, "Clinical Experiment in Secured Systems That Transforms Ventilation into Discrete Medical Treatment: Ethical Introduction." Report submitted to the Israeli Ministry of Health by the Chief Officer of Medical Ethics, February 2, 2002. sec. A3.

The Jewish Physician and End-of-life Decisions

Shimon M. Glick

A MONG THE MOST DIFFICULT situations any mortal can face is the prospect of death. The fear of death is universal, transcending cultures and eras.

No one has yet returned from death, and we all have difficulty in imagining an end to our own existence. This is an issue with which every society has to deal, each in its own way.

In the past century, the realities of death have been altered dramatically for the first time since the onset of human history. Scientific medicine and its attendant technology have for the first time provided tools that can clearly and obviously snatch individuals from the clutches of what in the past would have seemed to be inevitable impending death and restore them to health. As part of this achievement, these advances in medicine have also greatly prolonged the dying process and have enabled individuals to go through the throes of death, as it were, more than once. An entire literature of death experiences has emerged in which individuals who "died" but were resuscitated describe their experiences. No one, obviously, has succeeded in attaining the messianic prospect of חצנל תוומה עלב ("He will swallow up death forever"), as described by our prophets, but the successes of modern medicine in saving lives have at times created the illusion that the ultimate fate of death can be thwarted if only one makes a supreme effort. As a result, patients are sometimes subjected to what seems to them and their families to be prolonged undignified torture in heroic efforts to keep them alive against impossible odds and often against their wishes.

I have been in the medical profession over fifty years and have experienced the revolution in the ability of modern medicine to save lives in formerly fatal situations. Simultaneously I have witnessed marked attitudinal changes toward death, dying, euthanasia, and related topics.

What are the Jewish attitudes toward end-of-life care? In our era of pluralism, there are many voices that claim to speak for Judaism. Jews are dramatically overrepresented in the field of medicine in virtually every culture, but not everything that Jews do represents Judaism. The daily habits of ethnic Jews, people who are Jews in name only, and who do not base their actions on an understanding of the Jewish approach, should bear little weight on our discussion. Anyone of any Jewish persuasion who cares about what Judaism has to say must fall back on the traditional Jewish sources, beginning with the Torah, through the Talmud. and including the writings of contemporary scholars.

The Halakhah represents a unique continuum of guidance, both judicial and ethical, over several millennia, which has dealt with the issues of life and death as they present in daily life. In addition, Jewish scholars have not neglected the input from aggadic sources that enriches the halakhic discourse and often gives dramatic illustrations of the Jewish desiderata.

Unquestionably, the Jewish tradition places a value on life probably unequaled in any other culture. While belief in the hereafter (*olam ha-ba*) is a basic tenet of Judaism, life itself presents for the Jew an unparalleled opportunity to accomplish so much in every available moment of life on earth. The value of human life has been characterized as infinite, based on the mishnah in Sanhedrin that derives this evaluation from the observation that in the biblical tradition all mankind emerged from a single human being, Adam, and therefore every life has the potential of an entire world.[1] This infinity concept, initially proposed by the late Rabbi Yechiel Tikutzinsky, was popularized by the late Rabbi Immanuel Jakobovits, the founder of the term and the discipline of "Jewish medical ethics," and it has been widely quoted ever since.[2] I have referred to this valuable concept as a "mythology," but not in a pejorative sense, because I believe that the message of this concept of the supreme value of human life is indeed a pivotal value in Jewish thinking. But as a matter of daily practice we do not, and ought not, act in literal consonance with the concept that a moment of life is really identical in value with an eternity of life.

Because of the enormous value placed on human life, we are expected to spare virtually no effort to save human life, even for a short time. And conversely,the deliberate taking of a human life is considered one of the most grievous sins a person can commit. Not only is the active taking of human life a terrible crime, but the Jewish tradition also considers an abstention from saving a life as a serious offense. In contrast to the Western notion of individualism under which a person is not obligated to come to another's aid, the Torah specifically admonishes us: "Do not stand idly by your fellow's blood."[3] Allowing someone to die while taking a laissez-faire attitude is not acceptable either for a physician or for a layman.

Thus there is virtual unanimity that active euthanasia, even for a suffering human being who is imploring the physician to take action to terminate the suffering, is simply not acceptable. Shortening a patient's life by deliberate injection or other similar means remains murder even if life is shortened just by a few moments, and even if the intention is compassionate.

No less forbidden is suicide or assisted suicide. One has no more right to take one's own life than to take another's life. It has even been suggested that suicide is, in a way, worse than murder. A murderer has an opportunity for repentance after the deed, and indeed death itself is regarded as a mechanism of forgiveness. But the person who commits suicide forfeits the possibility of repentance, for the very act of death, which might redound to a person's credit, is in this case itself the result of a venal sin.

The Halakhah is strict about denying Jewish burial to those who commit suicide, and there are other strictures intended to put suicide out of the realm of social acceptability.

It is true that there are examples in the Bible and in Jewish martyrology of cases of suicide under a variety of extraordinary circumstances. In addition, rabbis often tried to be as lenient as possible with suicide victims so as not to cause further hurt to the bereaved families. Nevertheless, in the medical milieu there can be no countenancing of suicide or of physician-assisted suicide.

It is worth noting that in the first five years of the state of Oregon's assisted-suicide law, requests for suicide resulted mostly from a feeling that life was no longer worthwhile, rather than from pain and/or physical suffering.[4]

While human life is a major Jewish value, suffering is not valorized to the same extent as in some other cultures. Jewish sources teach us to accept suffering and describe it as having certain redeeming features. But unquestionably we are commanded to do our utmost to relieve the suffering of others. In fact, some Jewish sources clearly state that prolonged suffering is a fate worse than death. It follows that physicians are commanded and required to use all their resources to treat pain and suffering. The all-too-common fear that led physicians for decades to be stingy with pain-relief medications for fear of addiction or because of the threat to life from the side-effects of narcotics have little place in our tradition. Even at the risk of danger to life, the Jewish physician is mandated to provide maximal pain relief. Of course the provision of pain relief must not be used as a subterfuge for deliberate euthanasia by excessive doses of narcotics, as is too often the case, but pain relief must be provided. Interestingly enough, the most recent data indicate that the fears about the danger of adequate doses of narcotics have been greatly exaggerated, and adequate pain relief, rather than shortening life, may often lengthen it.

A fascinating insight into Jewish attitudes can be gleaned from the response to the question of whether one may pray for a suffering patient's death. While the usual situation is one of prayer for the patient's recovery, not infrequently one is faced with hopeless situations in which the patient is suffering greatly, and onlookers are tempted to pray for the patient's demise to relieve the suffering. Since prolonged suffering may be regarded as a fate worse than death, some Jewish sources permit prayer for a suffering patient's death.

The Talmud brings a most dramatic story about a sage who was suffering greatly from his illness.[5] His colleagues, all scholars like him, were praying for his recovery. But his devoted maid, who had witnessed the intensity of his suffering, prayed for the opposite, asking that he be granted death to relieve his suffering. In the symbolic tug of war, the poor maid stood no chance in heaven against the array of rabbis. But this simple woman took the initiative and smashed a pitcher; the noise startled the rabbis, interrupting their prayer, and so her prayer, now unopposed, triumphed, and the rabbi's suffering was ended by death.

That the text relates this tale without criticism suggests to some halakhic authorities that her act was meritorious.

More recently, a nineteenth-century rabbinical scholar, Rabbi Hayyim Palache, in Izmir, Turkey, was consulted by a devout layman about his wife, who had been incurably ill for many years and was now begging for an end to her life.[6] Active euthanasia, of course, was not even considered by this observant Jew, but he did ask his rabbi whether the Jewish tradition permitted prayer for his wife's death: this might be classified perhaps as a legitimate and merciful act of compassion. The rabbi responded with his usual scholarly erudition, compounded by thoughtful sensitivity to the couple's plight.

After a lengthy discussion, considering all aspects of the issue, he concluded that it was indeed permissible to pray for the sufferer's demise under these grave circumstances. But with great perceptive insight into human psychology, he restricted the prayers to individuals who were not directly involved in the care of the patient. Their prayers were sanctioned because their sole concern was the welfare of the patient. Family members, and other involved in any way in caring for the patient, were disqualified, because their prayers might have been tainted with a degree of self-interest. Perhaps they would be praying, to some extent, to be relieved from the burden the patient imposed upon them. This was a remarkably perceptive observation, and one in line with a long tradition in the Jewish legal system of disqualification of judges and witnesses for the slightest suggestion of even subtle unconscious bias.

In an era of increasing concern about the cost of health care and daily references to rationing it, one cannot help wondering whether some of the pressure for euthanasia in the Western world stems from considerations other then the welfare of the patient.[7] In the Jewish viewpoint, only the needs of the patient are the determining factor.

Although direct human intervention in life-shortening steps is precluded, the physician is permitted to withdraw or withhold certain treatments that are normally offered a patient who is not dying, but whose absence may hasten the death of a dying patient. Western medical ethics grants priority to the autonomy of patient and physician, and thus the patient is not obligated to seek medical care, and the physician is not obligated to render medical assistance. In contrast, under Jewish law both the physician and the patient have these obligations. Thus, theoretically at least, one might impose therapy on a competent patient who refuses it.

Nevertheless, the "fine print" of the Halakhah greatly restricts this possibility to treatments of absolutely proven effectiveness and no serious side-effects, a situation which rarely exists in the usual case of an end-of-life patient. Therefore, for all practical intents and purposes, the Halakhah allows dying patients to refuse even life-saving therapy if they do not feel the treatment worthwhile for their situation. We are permitted to gently persuade the patient to undergo treatment, but we may not apply inordinate psychological pressure and certainly not physical coercion.

The spectrum of treatments to be considered for withholding and/ or withdrawal is quite wide, ranging from cardiopulmonary resuscitation (CPR) to provision of nutrition and hydration. Cardiopulmonary resuscitation, introduced in the 1960s, was intended for the reversal of sudden death in relatively healthy individuals who suddenly developed an arrhythmia. It then began to be applied nonselectively to almost every patient who died in a hospital irrespective of the chances of success. Theoretically one can imagine an institution where everyone approaching death would be connected to a respirator and given cardiac massage to prolong life even for a few minutes, but this would be a perversion of medicine, common sense, and ethics. One of the reasons for the public pressure in favor of euthanasia was the excessive use of CPR, resulting in severe suffering and anguish to patients and their families.

In reaction to the overuse of CPR there developed the concept of DNR (do not resuscitate) orders which indicated which patient would be permitted to die without attempts at resuscitation. Under ideal circumstances, decisions about DNR orders should be made only after serious discussion among the staff, and involving the patient and family, rather then leaving the decision to a harried intern at 3:00 a.m. who does not know the patient and is likely to err in either direction. DNR decisions taken with due consideration of the likelihood of success, the potential side-effects, and the desires of the patient can be legitimate in Judaism. So too may one legitimately withhold life-saving therapy in a patient at the end of life if the patient decides to refuse therapy.

The more difficult, dangerous, and uncomfortable the therapy, the greater is the halakhic acceptability of the patient's refusing the therapy. In general we permit patients to refuse surgery, chemotherapy, dialysis, and almost any major therapy, even at the cost of shortening the patient's life. The greater the risk/benefit ratio, the less strongly will the physician attempt to persuade the patient to accept the suggested treatment.

The more difficult issue is the question of withdrawal of a therapy that has already begun. Over the past few decades, Western secular ethicists have by and large concluded that there is no fundamental difference between withholding therapy and withdrawing it. The intent behind equating these two approaches is clearly to relieve the hesitation of health personnel about withdrawing therapy by persuading them that it is no different from withholding therapy, a measure they have already accepted. Interestingly enough, however, the physicians and nurses who actually turn off the respirator or withdraw some other therapy are not so convinced of the ethicists' conclusion. The very same issue of the *Journal of the American Medical Association* in which an article stated that the notion of a difference between withholding and withdrawing therapy was a "myth"[8] reported on a poll of close to five hundred physicians working in premature nurseries in ten European countries showing that 66 percent of them did not see the two procedures as identical.[9]

I would call attention to the conceptual problem of lumping together markedly different psychological and practical actions under the rubric of withdrawal. Withdrawing a procedure such as dialysis, which is intermittent in nature, is much closer to withholding than is turning off a respirator for a patient who is totally respirator dependent. The nurse who turns off the respirator and see the patient die before her eyes moments afterward often cannot differentiate this act of hers from active euthanasia.

A further differentiation must also be made even in respect to a procedure like turning off a respirator. The inevitability of the outcome and the proximity of the outcome make an enormous difference. Turning off a respirator on a curarized patient with resultant 100 percent mortality within minutes is indeed a kind of active euthanasia. On the other hand, turning off the respirator on a patient who no longer can tolerate the intubation but may be able to be weaned from the respirator has entirely different implications. Karen Ann Quinlan lived for nine years after being disconnected from her respirator by court order.

The most difficult cases are those of patients with severe neuromuscular disorders whose life depends on a respirator but who insist on being disconnected. As described in Dr. Steinberg's article in this volume,[10] here too a solution has been developed whereby the cessation of the respirator is converted from a withdrawal of therapy, which is not acceptable according to most halakhic authorities, to a withholding of therapy, which under certain conditions may be acceptable.

At the other end of the spectrum is the patient who is brain dead by modern Western criteria. Here there is no suffering, and the issue is usually removal of organs for transplantation if the family consents. In this area there is a currently irresolvable conflict between two views in rabbinical circles. The Israeli Chief Rabbinate and several other leading authorities accept brain death if the standard criteria are followed strictly and if the clinical testing is confirmed by some objective test, such as intracranial Doppler testing. On the other hand, a significant number of haredi (ultra-Orthodox) halakhic authorities do not accept brain death as death and insist on cessation of heartbeat. In the view of the former decisors, all therapy may be stopped, and indeed should be stopped, to enable early burial of the body. On the other hand, the latter authorities would regard shutting off the respirator as an unjustified shortening of human life. Several of the contributors to this volume have dramatically and apparently irreconcilable differences of opinion on this critical decision.

In contrast to the conscious, competent patient, who, from most points of view, may almost never be coerced into accepting treatment, the patient who is comatose, or mentally incompetent, no longer has decision-making capacity. The decisions must then be made by others. We are obliged to act within the halakhic value system, which is clearly different from the currently prevailing views in many Western countries. The sanctity of life, a value deliberately excluded from the famous quartet of ethical principles emerging from Georgetown University, is dominant in Jewish thinking. Human life is not regarded merely instrumentally, in accord with its "quality." It has inherent value, even if this value is not obvious to outsiders. Therefore we would continue to treat a patient who is in a permanently vegetative state or who is suffering from incurable cancer until virtually the last throes of the patient's life. We would give antibiotics for pneumonia, insulin for diabetes, blood transfusions for anemia, and so on, even though there is no realistic chance for recovery from the basic state. Neither the family nor the physician has the right to decide that the life of a person in this condition is not worth living. Most authorities, however, would not insist on cardiopulmonary resuscitation if the patient went into cardiac arrest. The views of the family, while important as an indication of the patient's wishes, would not be determinative in stopping therapy. On the other hand, the clearly expressed, well-documented wishes of the patient could be given considerable weight in withholding some therapy from a patient who is suffering and near the end of life.

One of the areas in which there has been considerable change in practice in the West as part of the "slippery slope" since the Karen Ann Quinlan case is the area of nutrition and hydration. Over the past decade, several court decisions in the United States and the United Kingdom, as well as several professional organizations, have classified feeding by nasogastric tube or percutaneous endoscopic gastrostomy (PEG) as a medical procedure that may be withdrawn from a patient who is in a permanent vegetative state or severely demented. Such withdrawal is done with the clear intent of bringing about the death of the patient within a few weeks. Ironically, much of the literature supporting this practice speaks in a contradictory manner, stating that the placing of a PEG does not lengthen life, but nonetheless proposing withdrawal to shorten life! In the Jewish view, withdrawal of a feeding tube is akin to directly killing and cannot be countenanced. The societal pressures for such actions are growing rapidly, accelerated to a major extent by economic considerations, but are simply not in accord with Judaism.

The past few decades have witnessed what I would regard as an alarming change in medicine's attitude toward the value of human life. The initial excesses in the unthinking application of modern technology to unnecessarily prolong suffering led to a counter-reaction, with much lesser hesitancy, to shorten patients' lives. This counter-reaction has deepened and accelerated. Human life, once reverently regarded as sacred, is now considered more instrumentally, and lives are being shortened with relative ease by withdrawal of therapy, assisted suicide, and even active euthanasia in many societies.[11] The slippery slope in ethical behavior is dramatically demonstrated in this area. In contrast, the Jewish tradition, divinely inspired, tempered by centuries of experience, remains a stable source of guidance. This tradition is a beacon of compassion and sensitivity to human suffering together with respect for the sanctity of human life.

Notes

1. BT Sanhedrin 4:5.
2. I. Jakobovits, *Jewish Medical Ethics* (New York: Philosophical Library, 1959).
3. Leviticus 19:16.
4. K. Hedberg, D. Hopkins, and M. Kohn, "Five Years of Legal Physician-Assisted Suicide in Oregon," *New England Journal of Medicine* 348 (2003): 691.
5. BT Ketubbot 104a.
6. H. Palache, *Hikekei Lev* (Salonika, 1840; reprinted Israel: Book Export Enterprises, 1978), vol. 1, responsum 50.
7. D.P. Sulmasy, "Managed Care and Managed Death," *Archives of Internal Medicine* 155 (1995): 133.
8. A. Meisel, L. Snyder, and T. Quill, "Seven Legal Barriers to End-of-Life Care: Myths, Realities and Grains of Truth," *JAMA* 284 (2000): 2495.
9. M. Rebagliato et al., "Neonatal End-of-Life Decision Making: Physicians' Attitudes and Relationship with Self-Reported Practices in 10 European Countries," *JAMA* 284 (2000): 2451.
10. See above.
11. C.F. Gomez, *Regulating Death: Euthanasia and the Case of the Netherlands* (New York: Free Press, 1991).

Implementing Empathy at the End of Life

Maurice Lamm

Law and Feeling: Halakhah and Regesh

We live in two geographies; one is a compacted map of sharp-angled streets, the other is a map of rolling hills and unexplored forests. When we relate this to the handling of the ill, they are the geographies of cure vs. care, of repairing vs. healing, of pills and machines to relieve pain vs. personal warmth to mitigate suffering.

Caring for people at the end of life requires an understanding of the *masorah* ("tradition") of *halakhah* ("laws and customs") and the *masorah* of *regesh* ("feeling, sensitivity, caring, empathy"). The Jewish religious world understands a *masorah* of *halakhah* quite well; it is, after all, this tradition which guides all Jewish religious observance and is dominant in religious thought.

But few are familiar with Judaism's unwavering emphasis on the heritage of *regesh*. Many even believe that *regesh* is a contemporary invention, important but not imperative. They hold that it is not only an invention of a "californiated" soft ethic, but an intrusion on the body of Jewish tradition. A thousand years ago in Muslim Spain, the moral philosopher Bahya Ibn Pakuda wrote *Hovot ha-Levavot*, "The Duties of the Heart," but religious academia today still denigrates the *lev* ("heart") matters of Judaism. What has brought us to this thinking in our *haredi* (ultra-religious) style Orthodoxy is a subject for a whole set of volumes.

Rabbi Joseph D. Soloveitchik (1903–1993) taught, by word and action, that Judaism consists of both of these roots; that *regesh* (feeling) is not inferior to Halakhah (law) and is not a stranger to a religion. On the contrary, it is absolutely appropriate that God gave Jews, indeed all peoples living in a society in which interrelationships are paramount, health-oriented spiritual guidelines *mipnei darkei shalom*, "for the sake of leading tranquil lives."

For example, the structure of Shemoneh Esreh, one of the central Jewish prayers, is halakhically designed to be architecturally correct: every word is accounted for, the sequence of themes is precise and unmovable, and the times of its recitation are exact, down to the minute. This is a good example of the *masorah of* Halakhah (the tradition of the Law). Yet these elements are not all that is required in order to comply with the religious standard for this most important prayer. The Shemoneh Esreh is referred to as *avodah she-balev*, "the service of the heart": it needs to be suffused with spirituality, *kavanah* ("intent, direction") – in a word, a prayer that requires *regesh* ("feeling").

There are abundant examples where the *masorah of regesh* is paramount, such as mourning practices, the very definition of *simhah* ("joy"), and the sensitive mind-set when giving charity to the poor. Judaism was not addressed to disembodied souls, antiseptic academics, and other-worldly saints. It couches these *regesh* instructions *bi'leshon b'nai adam*, in familiar straightforward language, so as to convey the obligation of empathy and sensitivity to people whose hearts and minds are crammed with contradictions, complexities, and non rational notions, and who are possessed by worries about health, making a living, seeking solace, and building families. Clearly, the Torah and its commentaries are a wealth not only of laws and ethical imperatives, but of character and emotions, and they deal with appropriate as well as deviant behaviors. It is a fool's errand to ignore this fact, which requires no authoritative citations, but is common sense.

This is especially evident in matters surrounding death, when the unique *regesh* of Torah and mitzvot ("obligations") is a *sine qua non* prerequisite. The *regesh* of mourning practices is handled in Jewish literature with a brilliant perception into human needs (although I believe that it is not understood in its true depth today). But the *regesh* of pre-mortem, end-of-life existence is hardly touched. For one, the manner of death has been transformed in the last fifty years: people used to die catastrophic deaths, but today they generally die degenerative deaths. This gives the family more time with the terminally ill, and beckons them to understand the profound *regesh* of the altered circumstance, the sensitivities and strategies that can enable the dying to live fully until they actually die. The first imperative of Jewish life is to live – even when in the process of dying. To implement empathy we must plumb the Jewish experience with infirmity, discover ways of relieving the suffering of both the dying and the surviving, and sharpen our *regesh* by designing religiously informed strategies for conveying comfort in a devastatingly uncomfortable environment.

Relieving the Suffering
There are two sentences freighted with the most tragic overtones known to man: "We have done everything we can. Now you're in God's hands." These words trigger a hail of emotions, from anger to fear to jealousy to guilt, that rip open the innards of those who care but are helpless. From this moment until the advent of death, the terminal patient and his family experience the most painful and critical hours of their lives.

What follows are the bases for managing the terminally ill Jew, and then a number of real-life strategies of care, emanating from the Jewish understanding of *regesh*, which caregivers could use.

Dying is the juncture between time and eternity. It is twilight, *bein ha-shmashot*, not day, not night, when the sun sinks behind the horizon. Curiously, it is precisely at the end of day that the deep colors of day and night blend and swirl in broad strokes on the brush-painted sky. It is like the twilight of the trees in the fall, when the leaves burst with a palette of colors, bringing together the greens and yellows of summer and winter. In physical nature, twilight squeezes out the most brilliant and memorable of scenes, but in human nature, twilight is most often a gray, bleak mist that is swallowed up by the onrushing blackness.

Ideally, this should not be so. After the initial trauma, the dying should experience a stillness, a serenity, a coming-together of all of the events of life, a bottom line that makes everything add up, peace that until now they never knew. No longer the relentless pressure to "make it," the drive to possess more and more. No more reputation to earn; no impossible goals to reach; no petty power to be acquired; no glorious models to imitate; nobody to impress; no more games to play. Terminal patients know at last that the bitch-goddess of success makes a mockery of sincere striving. Finally, too finally, they can become detached from everything that is not truly an extension of their own self. They can love whoever they wish to love; no more ulterior motives. They are left with their mind and their soul and their memories and their faith and their values; and only with real friends and family. It may be the first time they can afford to live in purity, and in total honesty with their private self.

Yet these times may become intolerable – when the ticking of the clock is too loud, when family members are confused, erupting in anger at no one, blabbering incessantly but to no point, pouring sweetness-without-substance over a sick relative; when the patient does not know what to think, what to say, what to do, what is proper, mentally transfixed by questions without answers: "Why me? What now? Who will take care?"

The individual has no experience in dealing with such matters. Until a generation ago, death usually came too quickly for the victim to ruminate, and that is why, according to the Halakhah, the definition of dying (goses) is a process that takes at most three three days. Today, when people die from degenerative diseases, the process of dying is often extended for six months and more. Because people spend more time with the dying, they have more time to be frightened; the mystery becomes greater, the emotional complexities overwhelming. The dying person, like most people, is used to being in the company of family or friends at every major step of life. Now death will terminate all relationships with everyone. That is the great fear. The end-of-life patient will let go of the offering hands all around, and will proceed to the precipice of life slowly and alone.

It is not only that individuals have not dealt with this matter in any creative, significant way. The community has not even put the management of dying on its agenda. The Jewish community, which deals successfully with the daytime concerns of youth movements and old-age homes and family services and hospitals, and also with the night-time concerns of cemetery and free burial and conferences on grief, has never dealt with twilight. But dying is the crisis of life. One can die in fulfillment and with meaning; or in misery – filled with hate and jealousy. The confrontation with death is the greatest test of personality and of culture. May we abandon our people at this crossroads?

Just as a Torah scroll, used for holy purposes, retains its holiness even when it becomes religiously disqualified, so we humans, having been created with the sanctity of God's image, retain our dignity even in death when the image disintegrates. Human remains possess the same holiness that characterizes a disqualified Torah scroll. Thus one may not dishonor a corpse, just as one may not desecrate the scroll. In dying, as even in death, man retains the integrity of having been created in God's image.

In fact, this Torah view of human worth is the basis of social work. The Western religions, derived philosophically from a Jewish base, hold that all people – especially those who are sick and infirm, or too young to take care of themselves – are the subjects of social work practice.

This idea translates itself into practical behavioral application in Jewish law. For example, the Torah mandates speedy burial because it compares a dead human being to a king's wayward twin brother who is being hanged. When people pass by, they say: "There hangs the king." The brother's hanging reflects upon the dignity of the king. In much the same way, the rabbis reasoned, if we unnecessarily leave a human corpse to linger unburied, shame accrues to the King of Kings; man's image is God's "twin." So too the performing of a routine autopsy, except when needed to save life, runs counter to Jewish law, which says that not only the soul but the body of the person that contained the image of God is not to be unnecessarily disturbed.

Moreover, dying must be confronted as a new reality. Franz

Borkenau classified cultures as death-defying, death-accepting, or death-denying.

The Egyptian culture, against which the Israelites rebelled, built society around the glorification of death, symbolized for ages by the pyramids.

America has a death-denying culture. In an era of possible nuclear holocaust and of the graphic nightly portrayal of bloodshed on television, this is comically absurd. We deny death by diversion, stupefaction, a closing of the eyes, wishful thinking. We repress our fear of death by developing the art of embalming – berouging the dead to make them look alive; by having family sit separate from friends in the mortuary, by masking graves with green mats and consigning the burial to hired diggers. Indeed, we gladly consign the dying to specialists: the physician, the charge nurse, the private nurse, the rabbi, the convalescent home operator, and finally the mortician. Someone else is always there to handle the terrible reality. "We can't bear to see it," we say in self-indulging compassion.

But by history and by theology, Judaism is death-defying. Of all the forms of ritual impurity, the most severe defilement is caused by contact with a dead body. Contrarily, holiness is identified with life. We refer to a "God of life," and we are unable to accept a "dead god," whether it be Adonis or Jesus. Through the centuries the Jew has followed Dylan Thomas's prescription, "Rage, rage against the dying of the light," and our survival relates directly to this.

Not only does Judaism defy death, but, as a consequence of the sin of Adam, it literally refuses to consider death a natural phenomenon. It is, as Adin Steinsaltz terms it, "the disease of life." Death is a distortion; a perversion of the holiness associated with life. Man is to do battle against the "spirit of defilement," which, in fact, is a lifelong battle against death, considered to be the worst defect of this world. The climactic last phrase of the traditional funeral service is *bila ha-mavet la-netzach*, "May God swallow death forever." In the end of time, man will be victorious; death will be defeated. *Herpat amo*, "the shame of His people will He remove from the earth." This is not only a fond wish, it has become a mandate to Jews to struggle, when feasible, against the end which inevitably will engulf us all. This philosophy informs the obstinate Jewish refusal to give up on life even against the most insurmountable medical odds. It explains the profound reluctance to pull plugs and stop treatments.

But we must live our daily lives before the realization of that ideality for which we strive. The reality that in the end we will face death mandates our confrontation with the process of dying. The traditional Jew is expected to prepare for death. He often sewed his own shrouds, purchased a burial plot while he was in the blossom of life, wrote a will, arranged his funeral, and handled his own death as the necessary though ever-present evil that it is. Man must accept death after defying it to the last. But repressing the reality of death is an un-Jewish attitude, and our elaborate attempts to deny it are a religious absurdity.

In this sense, we are called upon to confront the reality of dying. In Jewish law, even such mundane matters as concluding a business contract and formulating a last will were guided by different, more binding and efficacious standards during these fateful days. This is a new reality, requiring new attitudes. It is not life as usual, and it is not the resignation of death. Hospice is effective to the degree that it looks upon the process of dying as a new stage of existence and uses different norms with which to realize our humanity.

Dying is not primarily a scientific event. Judaism makes a clear distinction between *bios* and *humanum*: physicality and humanity. It is important to determine at what point before birth the fetus goes from *bios* to *humanum*, from a simple physical organism to a fully developed human being; and at dying, at what point the *humanum* returns to *bios*, when one loses one's distinctive sanctity as a human being and becomes a vegetating organism. The Halakhah, for this reason, extends a person's *humanum* well beyond the conscious state until the last breath of existence as a person.

Judaism forcefully and legally affirms that a human being may never be treated solely as *bios*, even during the terminal process of dying. Man is not primarily a fact. Dying is not primarily a scientific event, it is a human one. During this period, the person has to be treated more humanely, more sensitively, not less.

The care given a dying person is a demonstration of whether the caregiver's emphasis is on *bios* or on *humanum*, halakhah or regesh. Judaism long ago established that it is concerned not primarily with sickness, but with the sick person. The Midrash says that even when there are only a few moments left to life, we should advise the dying person, "Eat this, drink that," notwithstanding that it cannot possibly make any difference. A deep concern for the prevention of human pain and suffering was uppermost in the rabbis' minds. Even when dealing with the angst of ordinary healthy people, all religious requirements are exempted in the face of pain. The Hebrew word for "doctor," *rofeh*, derives from the Hebrew word *rapeh*, which means "to ease" or "to assuage."

Hospitals, which treat *bios* exclusively, characteristically do not relate to a sense of shame on the part of the patient, to the need for privacy, personal delicacy, the need for warmth. The hospice, which emphasizes the *humanum* component and treats not only the illness but the patient, provides a team of psychologists, clergy, social workers, doctors, and nurses, but mainly family and volunteers, because it has a primary concern for human comfort and for the prevention and control of suffering.

The difference between an emphasis on *bios* and on *humanum* is tellingly illustrated in the style of informing patients of their terminality. One can announce it in a direct and accurate clinical diagnosis. But with an emphasis on the *humanum*, the telling can be a gradual self-revelation, a sort of Socratic self-understanding. After all, the shortest distance between two points is not necessarily a straight line when the straight line deals with a personal cataclysm, the upsetting of the whole natural order. If the patient chooses to deny the validity of the medical conclusion, Judaism tells us to respect his denial. Helmut Thielicke quotes a Japanese doctor who said, "There are lies that express profound human love." Truth we should tell, but the superior value is not truth but humanity. In all cases the old folk-wisdom obtains: "Be a mentsch" (Yiddish for "humane").

The care of the terminally ill, then, must embody certain fundamental principles: that we are created in the image of God and retain our integrity no matter who or in what condition we are; that a person's humanity should elicit from us sensitivity and delicacy; that defying death is an ideality and a hope, but the reality of our situation requires that we struggle to preserve life and, failing that, we struggle to preserve humanity, so long as we live. We were created as human beings; we must nurture that creation by being human.

Strategies for implementing Empathy
These underlying attitudes of the Jewish religion are expressed in specific strategies that ameliorate the agony attendant on a dying situation. If it is the true religion we believe it to be, Judaism must translate its moral axioms into policies of healthy behavior; virtually into a medicine-bag of attitudes which can make the twilight meaningful. These attitudes inform the Jewish component in hospice care. The Jewish part deals not only with the Halakhah of medical-cure ethics, but with the Halakhah of care ethics. As there is a Jewish way of living, so too there is a Jewish way of dying – and of caring for the dying. The rich Jewish heritage, which through the centuries has experienced man in the zenith of his growth and the nadir of his decline, has designed helping strategies for coping with the problems of the severely ill:

Loneliness
That the dying are lonely is of course understandable. The shock has thrown them back on theirs own resources. They will travel the road to their ultimate destiny wholly alone, without any company.

But they are lonely for two other reasons as well.

The dying have already begun to mourn themselves, their own death, the world that will go on without their presence, without their direction. In Hebrew, the word for "mourner" is *avel*, which means "one who withdraws." The family withdraw, and become *avelim*, after the dying patient's death, but the patient begins now to withdraw in mourning for himself.

The dying are alone not only because of their own psychological state, but because others cause them to suffer a pariah syndrome; they are figuratively placed outside the social pale. If death is a terminus of relationships, then dying is its prelude, and relationships now begin to become strained and to alter. It is like a candle flame about to be extinguished that flickers and sputters before it dies. Among the flickerings in personal relationships are the friends and relatives who shy away from the severely ill because they do not know what to say, how to express their genuine feelings of remorse. The patient, amputated from the living body politic, becomes passive, abandoned, and disconnected precisely when what is needed is connectedness to overcome the forbidding loneliness of dying.

Judaism addresses itself to this problem through the religious requirement of *bikkur holim*, "visiting the sick." The sick visitation is not merely a practice of social etiquette, but the fulfillment of a religious obligation. Unfortunately, the structure and content of this important function is very often not properly focused. It is simply an exercise in undiscerning sweetness – important, but not crucially helpful. We pay scant attention to what the tradition demands from this religious institution and how psychological findings can enrich it.

Visits should be frequent but of short duration, in keeping with the patient's fatigue threshold. We are not to hover over the bed, not to stand, but to sit on the patient's level. The patient is constantly looking up at doctors and nurses and visitors and made to feel like an object "over" whom people work. We must never leave without praying in the patient's presence. We must never leave without expressing hope (as described below).

The very presence of people is a therapeutic presence and considered a very great mitzvah ("obligation"). It reassures the patient of his continuing worth as an individual and reinforces the feeling of being an integral member of the family and the community. Traditionally, in fact, a minyan of ten Jews (the minimum number for a public service) was gathered to be present at the expected moment of life's expiration.

Apology

Jewish tradition understands that, in order to achieve a degree of inner peace, end-of-life patients need the process of *mehillah*, the asking of forgiveness from those they may have wronged. It is wiping the slate clean, an unburdening of the accumulated baggage of a lifetime. Indeed, they also need *mehillah* of another kind. Even though death is not an act of will on their part, many patients feel a need to apologize, and seek "permission," for leaving their families and for the pain they cause them by dying. The need may not be expressed openly, and in response it may require only a look of recognition, a holding of hands; but it should not be mocked or ignored.

Prayer

Maimonides rules that no *bikkur holim* visit is complete without prayer for the sick person. Prayer is considered a gift, not an obligation, and it can be a great comfort to many patients. There is formal prayer, recited from the prayerbook three times daily in the traditional manner. There is also informal prayer, which can be recited in any language, in any posture, at any time. This prayer may ask for an extension of life or for remission from pain. It also may be used to vent anger and complaint, even to ask for a rapid death. Prayer is especially valuable at this time because it allows for the articulation of hopes and fears in an accepted and elevated manner, and because it is offered as a communication from one who is powerless to the Almighty. Even those who do not customarily pray or even believe in God are often moved to do so in such conditions. "Pray for me" is a phrase often heard in hospital corridors. "Pray for yourself" is equally valid and even more helpful.

Curiously, the code of Jewish law suggests that whereas prayers recited in the synagogue or outside the room should be in Hebrew, the prayer in the patient's room may be recited in any language the patient understands. Prayer, in this sense, serves the twofold purpose of petitioning God and comforting the sick. It is also entirely proper and probably very comforting to the patient to recite a prayer for the sick in the synagogue before an open Torah scroll. This prayer is called Mi she-Berakh ("He who blesses").

Traditionally, over the centuries, the last syllables uttered by Jews as life nears its end are the words of a confessional prayer called

Viddui ("Confession"). It is a cumulative apology to God for the misdeeds of a lifetime. The sages considered it extremely valuable as an expiation for all sins. It is brief and moving. Great care should be taken to introduce this prayer delicately, assuring the patient that many have recited the prayer and survived. If it might traumatize the patient, it should not be recited. An abbreviated form of confession is as follows: *Teheyai mitati kapparah al kol avonotai* ("May my death be an atonement for all my sins"):

> I acknowledge unto Thee, O Lord my God and God of my fathers, that both my cure and my death are in Thy hand. May it be Thy will to grant me a perfect healing. Yet if Thou hast decreed that I should die, may my death expiate all the sins which I have committed before Thee, and grant me a portion in the Garden of Eden and cause me to merit the life of the World to Come, which is reserved for the righteous. Hear, O Israel, the Lord our God, the Lord is one.

Hope

What hope is possible for the dying? Yet, in the midst of this apparently hopeless situation, one is mandated by the Jewish tradition to inject hope into every visit, every conversation. But what can one hope for? Pessimists are fond of saying that from the moment of birth one proceeds every day closer to death. Helmut Thielicke observes that this is not quite true. He makes an analogy with walking. Every step we take seems to be a falling, and yet at the very last moment, before we really fall, we stretch forth our other leg and straighten up again. After a series of fallings and risings, we find that we have made progress through these ups and downs. But dying is, after all, the time of the final falling. What straightening up can come?

What rising sun can be expected from this twilight? Yet hope we must. One can hope for less pain, for the future happiness of children, for the family's continuation of the values one has spent a lifetime instilling. While there should be an intelligent awareness of hope's limitations in this situation, a sincere expression of hope is required by the tradition. In fact, Jews believe that death may be the beginning of exaltation, a reunion of the divine image with the divine source of being, as Abraham J. Heschel says:

> Death is not sensed as a defeat but as a summation, an arrival, a conclusion. Our ultimate hope has no specific content, our hope is God. We trust that He will not desert those that trust in Him. The meaning as well as mode of being which man hopes to attain beyond the threshold of dying, remains an impenetrable mystery, yet it is the thought of being in God's knowing that may be both at the root and the symbol of the ultimate hope.

Here follows an illustrative case history:

> Dr. Alexandra Levine at the University of Southern California (USC) Medical School reports an experience as a medical student. A 55-year-old woman was admitted to the hospital with a lesion in the right lung. She was not in pain, and was affable and very cheerful and helpful to the health personnel on the floor. She was transferred to surgery for an open thoracotomy, and was found to have squamous cell carcinoma that had metastasized and was inoperable. Then a section was removed for biopsy and the incision was closed.
>
> She had to be informed of the terrible news. The resident entered the room with a gaggle of interns behind him, stood at the bed, looked down at her, and had this conversation with her.
>
> Resident: Well, it's cancer and we couldn't really resect it, so we just opened and closed.
> Patient: Opened and closed?
> Resident: Yes, well, it couldn't be removed, so we just closed. It was useless.
> Patient: Opened and closed?
> Resident nodded.
> Patient: Opened and closed?
> Resident nodded again.

Patient: You mean you left the cancer there?

Resident: Yes

The patient died that night. The autopsy showed no actual cause of death, just the cancer, which had been there for many months. Dr. Levine writes in the *Western Journal of Medicine* that she believes the patient simply died out of despair, the removal of esperanto, HOPE, all hope had been squeezed out of her.

Comment:

1. The resident de-hoped the patient. He did it with words, with body language, with unthinking and callous disregard.

a. He should not have brought a squad of interns when he was to tell a person that she is going to die. Does anything more critically deserve privacy than this event?

b. He should not have stood next to her bed, he should have sat down. First because a person lying down feels more vulnerable when somebody stands over her. Second because he looks like he has to get out of there fast, and can't afford the time to stay.

c. He de-hoped her by saying nothing could be done. She had the pain and the scar and nothing was done? He never mentioned that other treatments could be tried.

2. How could the resident have en-hoped her?

a. Without lying he could have said that some of the tumor was removed, though not all of it.

b. That further therapy would be required to attempt to deal with the remainder.

c. He could have said that miracles happen every day and that she might be one of them.

d. He could have told her that researchers are coming up with new medications, and who could tell whether she could be lucky enough to get a working remedy.

e. Also he could have used the old medical escape, "It's in God's hands. I pray that He will help you."

Would he have saved her life? Ultimately no. Would she have lived longer? This lady died too soon of evident heartbreak. Hope might have enabled her to live while she was dying.

Power

Dying patients find themselves in a passive condition. They are power-less to initiate significant actions or make significant decisions. They are tested and turned and injected; they are cried over and spoken behind and prayed for. They have effectively been removed from the dynamic world. The Jewish tradition provides for specific activities which give them a sense of power – thoughts to be managed, projects to be executed which can excite the mind and spark one's imagination to think creatively, even during this time of smallness.

Ethical wills. In order to give them some initiative, terminal patients should be encouraged to write an ethical will. This is an ancient Jewish device. People should leave their families not only an estate but also a heritage. Sometimes parents have not been able to communicate effectively with a child or grandchild. This affords them opportunity to leave their loved ones a sense of their purpose in life, their values and beliefs, in a format that will be treasured after death.

Oral history. Another application of empathy which is of clear value at this time is leaving behind the legacy of an oral history. By speaking into a tape-recorder to be transcribed later, patients can give living roots to their families. They can tell where they were born and what their parents were like, they can give an account of their youth and education, of their beliefs and dreams. A mate, child, or nurse can assist by asking pertinent questions and guiding the conversation. Describing one's life in this way invokes good feelings, both in recalling pleasant memories during the days of recording the personal history, and then in giving children a gift volume describing their family roots. It is little short of an intimation of immortality.

Charity. The Jewish sages said that "Charity rescues from death." Obviously the sages were not speaking of magic. They meant that it saves the dying from the feeling of death. Distributing charity, no matter who the recipient or what the amount, and deliberating on who should receive it, may give a person a feeling of strength and a sense of being alive.

Setting one's house in order. The time of dying is a time to make arrangements for one's family, and for dealing with one's own personal attitudes and status and relationships. The patriarch Jacob was blessed with illness, the rabbis say, in order that he might prepare for death. The prophet Isaiah tells King Hezekiah: "Set thy house in order, for thou shalt die, not live"

Reminiscence

Virtually all terminally ill people prefer to die at home rather than in an institutional setting, even a caring, free-standing hospice. This is not only because of the personal care and the presence of family members, but also because the home surroundings are familiar and a source of security at a time of fearful uncertainty.

This universal sentiment is the origin of a number of traditions. Among them is that in the last hours of life the dying should be surrounded by a minyan of people, akin to the quorum required for public prayer. Death too is a moment of sanctity, as is a prayer service.

But it is also an awareness that the ambience of friends and relatives makes for warmth and a great relief from the fear of loneliness.

The terminally ill desperately desire what they know they cannot achieve, life, getting out of the bed, back to the old days. Reminiscence is really episodic recall. We change the ambience of those who are sick and enable their minds, even if only for a short time, to fly away from their troubles to an earlier, healthier time.

Neuroscientists hold that the human mind is like a tape-recorder, stacked with an infinite number of dormant memories. Recalling these long-forgotten memories is like digging up subcortical imprints of remote events. With the collaboration of the patient, we rewind the tape, and the scenes fly by as we focus on another era. The content of this episodic recall is triggered by soft words from sympathetic eager-to-listen relatives and friends. It is a vacation from the constant bad news of the current situation – vacations, celebrations, heroic achievements, incidents that stirred pride, weddings and births and grandchildren, a Bar or Bat Mitzvah, long-dead relatives, another country, a happier time. One of the qualities of the human brain is that, even though the senses are fading, it has the ability to soar back to old scenes for instantaneous recall.

This iconic replay of life's repertoire can transform a patient's mood more humanely than mind-altering drugs. The God-given capacity to forget events too horrific to deal with can now be abetted by the God-given function of remembering.

Love

Since time is now limited, life becomes ever more precious, and the relationship between the family and the dying person should be intensified in depth and quality. This should be a period when loved ones sustain and cherish the patient. Perhaps the relationship has been strained for many years, that there were dissonances and bickering, and t therefore that the expression of love now suddenly demonstrated is felt to be hypocrisy. But now life is new and love can begin anew. Rabbi Eliyahu Dessler, the twentieth century's greatest Jewish ethicist, asks: Which comes first – giving or loving? The common answer is that one gives to a person whom one already loves. But the reverse is also true. One loves the person to whom one has given. The more parents give to a child in need, the more the love grows.[10]

At a time of terminal illness, the family should give of themselves. They should hug and stroke and touch the patient. The giving may exalt love to a level that was hitherto unimaginable.

The art of loving is most strained when you love someone who is approaching death. Done properly, love can rise to its most intense level at precisely this moment; feelings can become more authentic than at any other time in life; the capacity for giving and for sheer goodness can be unimaginable, and their effect can physically lengthen a person's life and make the last moments beautiful. These last expressions of love plumb our deepest personal resources.

A friend of mine, Jack Goldberg, was trying to impel his wife, Mary, to take more medicine in her dying days. He said to her, "Mary, I'm not giving you poison." Mary looked at him and said. "Jack: I never thought you were capable of caring for me so much. Even if you gave me poison, from you I would take it as medicine."

It is twilight. As the sun falls behind the horizon, human life, like nature, can produce a burst of color – the color of meaningfulness, of hope and love.

Ethics and Reality

AN ISRAELI NURSE'S PERSPECTIVE

Lydia Goldschmidt

T HE SOUND of a siren at 2:00 P.M. on October 6, 1973 invaded the
silence of Yom Kippur, the highest Jewish holiday. I was expected
at the hospital as a staff nurse in the neurology department at four
o'clock, but the breaking news about the war that had started a few
hours earlier urged me to put on my uniform and hurry to the hospital.
We could feel the sense of stress and disaster in the air. As a nurse
who had just completed her formal professional education, I did not
fully understand that these days would shape my whole perspective
as a nurse and as a human being forever.

When I entered the ward, a senior doctor was already there. Together we made a quick assessment of the patients and decided which
of them to send home in order to empty the ward, since it was quite
obvious that the beds would soon be filled with wounded soldiers. It
was not until many years later that I understood that the decisions
we made in those days were very difficult clinical-ethical decisions.
Even today I still wonder whether the discharge of the thirty-four-
year-old patient who had a tracheotomy only a couple of days before
was the right decision. At the time I was too young and inexperienced
to ask.

The next day I was transferred to the respiratory intensive care
unit (RICU) and served there until the hospital was back to normal six
months later. Nothing could be compared to this period and the many
dilemmas we faced, and nothing afterwards seemed difficult anymore.

Life and death, teamwork, intensity of work were not phrases – it was our reality at that time.

One of the ethical decisions imposed on us during the war was the need for intensive care beds. Most of the senior doctors were either in the operating room or were mobilized in the army. The nursing staff functioned under the supervision of a first-year anesthetist and a fifth-year medical student. On my first day there, we were notified that a severely wounded soldier was on the way who needed to be admitted to the RICU. The question was, Who would have to be transferred out, and whose chances of survival outside the unit were best? All of the patients needed respiratory support, but each of them had an additional social component that had to be quickly taken into consideration. One of the patients was a respected contributor to the hospital, another was a well-known rabbi, the third was a nurse at the hospital, and one was a member of the hospital's executive committee. The fifth bed was occupied by a five-year-old Arab child who was suffering from polio, completely paralyzed, and dependent on a respirator, and had been abandoned by his family. I don't remember the decision-making process, but I still remember the decision. The child was sent to the children's department with the respirator. I heard he died a few weeks later. Thirty years and several wars later, and with the knowledge of how many lives the RICU had saved at the time, I still ask myself: Was it the right clinical decision? Was it an ethical decision?

These experiences led me to the field of nursing ethics, a subject I deal with in my daily practice as a nurse, teacher, and nursing administrator. Based on my experience, the ethical problems and dilemmas encountered by nurses in Israel can be divided into three groups:

1. *Responses to specific events*. These may result from two factors.
a. *Personal background*. Israel is a small country. People know each other from school, military service, university, and other social circles. When there is a terrorist attack, one thinks automatically that a family member or a friend may be hurt. More than half a year ago, this was one of the questions asked while treating casualties from the suicide

bombing in Café Hillel, when the head of the emergency room (ER) did not show up. He always came early, even before the first ambulance arrived. This time he was one of the victims. We learned a few hours later that he and his daughter had been killed in the attack; it was just a day before the daughter's wedding.

b. *Religious and political views*. Nurses in Israel are taught to treat patients without regard to their political affiliations. This can be quite difficult when the patient is definitely from a different social, ethnic, or political group. In the seventies, two Arab students were preparing a bomb in the dormitories of the Hebrew University in Jerusalem. The bomb exploded in their hands, and they were brought to the ER along with innocent casualties. One of the bombers was a beautiful young female student, with long black hair. She was brought in covered with blood and metal fragments. There were two of us who treated her – an Orthodox nurse and me. She wanted to cut the girl's hair, I thought it would be a breach of her autonomy. Finally, weeping together, we both washed the blood and metal from the girl's hair.

2. *Influence of financial considerations and legislation on ethical problem-solving in hospitals and community settings*

3. *Changes in nursing, nursing education, and professional development, and in the interdisciplinary relationship between nurses and doctors.* These developments led to more consideration of nurses' opinions regarding the condition and treatment of patients, such as hydration in end-of-life situations. Nurses tend to favor restricting hydration, because hydration makes a dying patient uncomfortable. Oncology nurses point out that the patients refrain from eating and drinking because it causes them pain.

These three kinds of factors may influence the process of decision-making concerning patient autonomy, sanctity of life, dignity of life, palliative care, or assisting suicide. Israel has experienced a wave of terror in the last three years which has confronted every one of us with difficult dilemmas regarding the end of life, not only with patients dying from disease, but often with critically injured young patients. It was no longer a theoretical debate about euthanasia of a patient slowly dying from disease. There were severely injured people who needed our decisions, who had been attacked and injured simply because they were Jews. The first responses came automatically: first aid, quick treatment in order to save life, no matter who the patient or caregiver was. Only later were we flooded by our emotions. The Orthodox Jewish nurse who was educated to save lives because life is sacred, who treated a woman injured in a suicide bombing – with a completely smashed face, no ears, the whole body broken and burned – asked herself: Is this suffering justified? Where is the limit? Does this severe suffering and the certainty of death justify prolonging life by all means? A very difficult ethical-moral-economical-human question.

Nursing of the dying patient and the Israeli code of Ethics

In Israeli hospitals the issue of the end-of-life patient is usually approached in a holistic way, trying to combine preservation of life with the principle of patient autonomy, always keeping the patient's interest in mind. Dealing with these questions, whether in hospital, the community, or nursing school, it is important to use precise terminology to define the nurse's role with all its practical and legal implications.

Physician-assisted dying (PAD) is a process whereby the nurse actually aids in ending a patient's life by executing the physician's orders, which implies that the nurse accepts the action. This kind of active euthanasia is not legal in Israel. PAD also contradicts the 1995 guidelines of the American Nursing Association (ANA), which focus on using modern technology and know-how to alleviate suffering and relieve pain at the end of a patient's life. A survey found that religious nurses approve more easily of PAD, but would not themselves administer any drug that will shorten a patient's life.[1] The same study also shows that Israeli nurses are more concerned with relieving a patient's pain and suffering than with the ethics of PAD.

Nurse-assisted dying (NAD) is the ending of a patient's life by a nurse with or without the patient's request, and without a doctor's order.[2] This is strongly opposed by the ANA because it is against its code of ethics. In Israel NAD is prohibited and is not even discussed publicly.

The Israeli code of ethics, which was written by nurses and for nurses in 1994, serves our nurses as a moral and professional compass on three levels: (1) professional relationships with patients, (2) relationships between nurses and society, and (3) relationships between nurses and their professional community.

The Israeli code of ethics deals with such issues as human dignity, quality and safety of life and of treatment, trust, social health, quality assurance, promotion and preservation of health, professional loyalty and mutual respect, freedom for professional struggle, nursing responsibilities, and the patent's right to privacy. The end of life care touches all three levels, although the code of ethics deals mainly with the nurse as an individual treating the patient as an individual.

The code values highly a person's dignity in life and death. Patients have the right to receive treatment without prejudice of religion, nationality, race, age, gender, political views, social status, or health, but their social background should also be considered in deciding on a treatment approach, because affiliation to a social or religious group may be relevant to a patient's end-of-life decision. The nurse must accept this background, and must explain it to the rest of the staff if the patient wishes her to do so.

Patients have the right to die with dignity in accordance with their own values. This may create a conflict between the patient's values and those of the family and friends or the medical staff. According to the code of ethics, the nurse should fulfill as many as possible of the dying patient's wishes, and help the family to cope with the loss. Fulfilling these rights and wishes can sometimes clash with the rights of other patients or their family members.

A somewhat bizarre situation sometimes occurs in Jewish hospitals. According to the Halakhah (Jewish religious law), when a person dies, people who are descendants of the biblical priests (*kohanim*) are not allowed to be in the building until the body is removed. If the deceased's family wants the body placed in the *taharah* room (where the body is ritually washed before burial), *kohanim* who are family members of other patients cannot enter the building until the usual warning sign is removed. This expresses the complexity of trying to preserve one's autonomy in the reality of a general hospital.

If a nurse is required to act against her own moral views or beliefs, she should pass on the treatment of the patient to another staff member, as in the case of DNR (do not resuscitate) orders. Agreement or disagreement with DNR depends on one's personal and professional point of view.

When executing a doctor's order which may shorten the patient's life, the nurse often feels as though she is the one who is causing the death. There is an emotional difference between approving the giving of drugs that may hasten death and performing the actual act of administering the drug, even if we use terms like "terminal sedation" (TS). Nurses feel that in performing the act of TS they betray the patient's trust in violation of their code of ethics.

Lacking uniform national guidelines, hospitals in Israel differ in their attitude toward dying patients. While one hospital will allow TS by ignoring it, another will fight for the patient's life at all costs with no regard for the patient's request or the caregiver's opinion. One hospital in Israel has published written instructions on DNR for its staff members that make the process more acceptable and easier to handle.

An important question is whether there is a fundamental difference between withholding treatment and withdrawing it, because in Israel withdrawing is considered active euthanasia and thus illegal. Although both achieve the same result, most caregivers feel there is a distinct emotional difference between the more passive involvement of withholding treatment and the more active role of withdrawing a treatment that has already been given. Another question is whether withholding treatment is not actually active euthanasia, since it is an active action in its own right resulting from an active decision not to prolong life.

Nurses in Israel will not actively participate in PAD because of this emotional difference. Being passive makes them feel less guilty about causing the patient's death and look less like "murderers in a white coat."

Nurses' organizations in Israel and the United States see the relationship between nurses and patients as a system of obligations mediated by a professional approach. This professional approach is based on mutual trust. Therefore, when debating end-of-life issues, both sides should consider all aspects to keep this fragile trust.

Kopala introduced the notion of ranking values.[3] The values of the patient that lead to the patient's decisions should be compared with the values of the nurses. The idea is to create a common ground between patient and caregivers which compares the patient's wishes with the possibilities for the caregivers to satisfy these wishes. If the patient's wishes are to be followed, there is a need to create precise directives for the caregivers.

Advanced medical directives (AMD) are accepted only in a few countries. They are not yet legal in Israel, but when they are accepted there, legal emphasis should be given to the nurse's responsibility in fulfilling the patient's wishes, patient dignity and autonomy, and the right of patients to decide on a course of action regarding the value of life as they see it, without causing caregivers to interfere with the sanctity of life. As in many other countries, nurses in Israel do not have the right to interfere with the patient's decision-making process regarding AMDs or DNR orders, in order to refrain from reaching a slippery slope and not stretching the limits of decision-making at the end of life with old, exhausted patients and the chronically ill who are not terminal. We try hard not to begin with the idea of the patient's right to die with dignity and end up with an obligation to die, being guided by immoral considerations such as costs or workload.

A hospice is an institution where people go to die. Dying patients admitted to a hospice know their diagnosis and prognosis (which is shorter than six months), have already gone through all the available tests and treatments with no chance of cure, and enter with the knowledge that they will not be subjected to forced feeding, drinking, or other life-saving measures if they so choose. A patient not accepted in a hospice due to lack of beds may end up in any other department of a general hospital, where there is no choice about eating and drinking and refusing life-saving measures. As a result, there may be a place for the hospice approach not only in the hospice itself but also in certain departments of general hospitals. This will allow us to preserve the dying patient's autonomy and dignity even thought the patient is not in a hospice.

Nursing in Israel and the Law

Nursing in Israel is legally not an independent profession, since it is practiced under The Doctor's Act (for community nurses since 1981, for hospital nurses since 1988). Although nurses are free to decide on and independently execute certain actions, in most instances they must follow the doctor's orders. Most medical-clinical orders do not entail conflicts between nurses and doctors. But conflicts may very well occur when the orders are of a mixed medical-clinical and ethical-moral nature. Contradictions may appear between the patient's wishes and the views of the patient's family, the doctors, or the nurses. Moral problems in nursingmay derive from the doctor's orders as well as from the nurse's feeling of professional inferiority. Orders that go against a nurse's conscience or professional understanding may be problematic for her to execute.

In the year 2000 the Israel minister of health appointed Prof. Avraham Steinberg to form a committee with the aim of setting guidelines in the form of a law proposal to guide everyone involved with dying patients. Elsewhere in this book Professor Steinberg gives a full account of the work of the committee and the resulting law proposal. I will just mention a few important points:

- A large committee was formed representing as wide a spectrum of society as possible, including physicians, philosophers, ethicists, psychologists, nurses, social workers, lawyers, and religious authorities from every faith in Israel (Jews, Muslims, Druse, Christians). The committee's aim was to create a fair equilibrium between the two principles of preserving life and respecting the patient's autonomy at the end of life.

- The emphasis is principally on preserving life and improving its quality in the dying patient by proper palliative means. The patient's autonomy to chose or avoid treatment should be respected as far as legally possible. Advance medical directives will be legal when written according to well-described guidelines. Physicians and nurses will be allowed to counsel patients in setting up an AMD in accordance with the patient's wishes and to provide the necessary medical information.
- With unconscious patients, the views of family or close friends will be taken into consideration.
- A caregiver who adheres to the rules of this legislation cannot be charged in any court for treating or not treating an end-of-life patient.
- Nurses will be considered equal staff members in the decision-making process.
- In unclear situations and when the caregivers, the patient, and the patient's family differ, the case will be brought before an ethics committee on which there is a nurse member along with doctors, social workers, psychologists, ethicists, and lawyers. Nurses will also have the authority to submit a request on their own or on a patient's behalf to an institutional or a national ethics committee.

This means that nurses in Israel should adopt a professional and personal view of the subject. An Australian inquiry among two thousand nurses showed that 66 percent of them were willing to take part in active euthanasia if it were legal.[4] Another survey conducted in Israel found that 72 percent of the nurses and 63 percent of the doctors in the community supported the legalization of euthanasia.[5] This finding pertains not just to the last few days in the life of a patient but frequently to several months. In Israel the end-of-life patient is defined as a person whose life expectancy is less than six months. Nurses would like to be partners in the process of decision-making with the end-of-life patient because they are with their patients in the hospital, the community, and,the hospice most hours of the day, if not all. The perception that doctors will give medical dictates to nurses during this long process is unacceptable, because they are the ones who have to work with the patients. Nurses see themselves as the patients' advocates, and giving help especially to disadvantaged patients, such as the elderly, ICU patients, AIDS patients, and the mentally disabled (retarded, demented). In all probability the nurse will act, if possible, in accordance with the wishes of adult patients who can express their wishes. Sometimes the nurse's personal views collide with the patient's wishes, and in such cases she will probably act according to her own beliefs, not those of the patient. The law proposal of the Steinberg Committee provides an answer for collisions of this kind by allowing the nurse to pass the job of caring for such a patient to another staff member who agrees with the patient's wishes.

Nurses are taught that death is a part of the life cycle. Within this cycle, the nurse will accompany her patients and support them in their decisions even if they chose not to keep on living. She will stay with them because this is what is expected of her profession. Staying with a dying patient is the heart of nursing and caring.

In the past, treatment decisions for end-of-life patients were generally made by doctors and approved by family members. Today those decisions should be made by the patient and whoever the patient chooses to participate jointly in the decision-making. Family members are not automatically a part of the decision-making process, and information about the patient's illness is not given to them without the patient's approval. It is the patient's right to decide how and when to die, not only because he is a patient, but because he is a free human being.

A nurse who chooses to restrict this human right because her personal religious beliefs treat life as the supreme value comes into conflict with the notion of patient autonomy. The right to be, the right to live, is a basic and universal human right. The law proposal of the Steinberg committee assumes that a human being *a priori* wants to live. But sickness and the terminal state may induct a patient to think otherwise and to wish to die. The right to die (with dignity) is therefore not self-evident, although the patient's wishes are morally justified. Nurses should help their patients to realize this right, not only because patients are often unable to hasten their deaths by themselves, but also out of compassion. Most nurses in Israel would be willing to participate in PAD if it were legal, but most would prefer to stay with the patient until the patient dies but have someone else administer the drug that will end the patient's life. A community nurse once phoned to tell me that one of her cancer patients, who had an IV morphine set at home, had asked his family during her visit to set the drip faster so that it would shorten his life. She stayed with him together with his family until he died.

Professional Education of Nurses

Since nursing is rapidly developing into an autonomous profession, nurses in the community as well as in hospitals face more and more dilemmas like the one mentioned above. As partners in the decision-making process, they should carefully consider these serious questions not only as individuals but also as professionals, taking into consideration the special situation of being a nurse in a state that is Jewish and democratic.

In Israel there are two different training courses for nurses, a shorter course for practical nurses (PNs) and a longer course for registered nurse (RNs). Since the 1970s there has also been an academic curriculum for nursing. RNs are permitted to choose to study higher professional education and expertise in courses like oncology, dialysis, trauma, intensive care, gerontology, and other fields. There has been a parallel growth between patients' autonomy and nurses' autonomy as expressed in the Israeli patient's bill of rights and the Israeli nurse's code of ethics. Nurses are taught not only to help patients clinically, but also to take part in the decisions of the care-giving team where they support the patient's interests. They are able to make assessments of the patient's needs because they usually have a closer relationship with the patient and family than other members of the staff. Nursing has changed since the early twentieth century, when the principal aim was to treat newborn babies, women after birth, and infectious diseases. Now, in the early twenty-first century, nurses are proficient with very complicated treatments and in the management of sophisticated modern equipment. Their education in problem-solving makes them partners in the decision-making process.

Today nurses also learn to make economic evaluations in the health services and participate in discussions and decisions about cost-effectiveness. As the administrator of the nursing division of a hospital, I am approached by nurses who are worried by these dilemmas. Many old patients are sent to the ICU and put on respirators. The nurses know that Judaism makes no distinction between young and old in deciding whether to connect a patient to a respirator. But they feel that it is an expensive and often ineffective and futile treatment. Putting an old man on a respirator may be the moral thing to do from the standpoint of the patient and family, but if financial resources are limited, wouldn't they better spent on a younger patient with more chance for survival?. Sometimes patients are even put on a respirator against their will or the will of their families – a fact which nurses are aware of but which is often disregarded by other staff members.

We must not forget that in Israel, as in other countries, the death of a patient can be a controversial economic issue, for it is less expensive not to put a patient with minimal chances of survival on a respirator. This is not a slippery-slope moral argument, but a practical managerial one, such as a lack of available respirators or shortage of specialized staff. When participating in making decisions of this kind, nurses must take care not to yield to irrelevant organizational considerations and to always keep the patient's interest in mind.

End-of-life decisions are crucial to how patients spend their last days and how they die. But the way decisions are made, balancing sanctity of life, autonomy, and dignity is no less important than the decision itself, both for the caregivers who make the decisions and for the profession they represent.

Because of Israel's unique geographical location, political and military situation, and demographic environment, its nurses – some with strong religious beliefs – are challenged daily by moral and ethical decisions not faced by nurses in other countries. Among these dilemmas are situations similar to the tracheotomy patient and the Arab child with polio from 1973 mentioned at the beginning of this article, and the woman with a totally smashed face who died in a suicide bombing thirty years later in Jerusalem in 2003. These horrible events make the decision-making process in relation to dying patients very difficult and emotional, but nonetheless necessary because human life is so valuable. As nurses and nursing educators, we must try to achieve a balance between the sanctity of life and the patient's wishes in order to preserve this valuable gift called life.

Notes

1. C. Mosgrave, I. Margalith, and L. Goldschmidt, "Israeli Oncology and Non-Oncology Nurses' Attitudes toward Physician-Assisted Dying: A Comparative Study," *Oncology Nursing Forum* 28, no. 1 (2001): 50–57.
2. J.K. Schwartz, "Assisted Dying and Nursing Practice," *Image: Journal of Nursing Scholarship* 31, no. 4 (1999): 367–373.
3. B. Kopala and S.L. Kennedy "Requests for Assisted Suicide: A Nursing Issue." *Nursing Ethics* 5, no. 1 (1998): 16–26.
4. S. Van Hooft, "Bioethics and Caring," *Journal of Medical Ethics* 22 (1996): 83–89.
5. I. Margalith, C. Mosgrave, and L. Goldschmidt, "Physician-Assisted Dying: Are Education and Religious Beliefs Related to Nursing Students' Attitudes?" *Journal of Nursing Education* 42, no. 2 (2003): 91–96.

Assisted Death?

SOME CLARIFYING PROPOSITIONS

Hans Küng

A Personal Preface

Speaking here as a theologian and as a Christian person, I am developing ideas which I presented back in 1994 together with my colleague and friend Walter Jens at the Tübingen Studium Generale and then published under the title "Menschenwürdig sterben" (Dying with Dignity). With Walter Jens's consent, I shall now start out from that rational "plea for personal responsibility," with the purpose of helping others, not only many patients but also doctors and judges, to clarify their ideas. Walter Jens and I wish to speak out on behalf of the innumerable unnamed patients whose stories have affected us deeply. Their individual fates, often unbearable, should not be smothered in lofty ethical, legal, and theological debate on fundamentals. For their sakes I, as a theologian, would like to develop an alternative and responsible path, based on my thinking over three decades.

1. In Christian belief, human life is ultimately God's gift, and is surely not owed by Man to himself. At the same time, life according to the will of God is also Man's duty. As such it has been placed at our responsible disposal (and not of others!). This holds true too for that final stage of life which is dying. Assisted death is thus to be understood as the final assistance to living, an expression – for the believer – of an autonomy grounded in theonomy.

Some say that every human being must hold out to "the ordained end" and must not give back his life "prematurely." But the good Creator nowhere "ordained" the reduction of human life to purely biological and vegetative existence; the free and responsible return, under unbearable suffering, of a life definitely destroyed is not "premature." Death is not always Man's enemy.

2. Incurable disease, the infirmity of old age, or final unconsciousness does not turn a human being into a "nonperson" or a "no-longer-human."

This deeply humane standpoint must be espoused against certain advocates of actively assisted death, such as the Australian moral philosopher Peter Singer. It is understandable that the severely handicapped in particular react strongly against this concept (indeed, sometimes excessively against any discussion of it). Basically there is no such thing as "a life not worth living." Singer's theses require a publicly debated rebuttal.

3. It is because humans are human and remain so to the end, whether mortally ill (death expected in the foreseeable future) or dying (death expected shortly), that Man has the right not only to a life of human dignity but also to a humanly dignified farewell and death. The hospice movement deserves moral support and practical social promotion, for here medical endeavor and therapy have yielded the center of the stage to personal attention through conversation and to endeavors affording a dignified death.

Not in every case does the right to go on living mean a duty to do so. Quite possibly, the right to a humanly dignified death is being denied to a person through indefinite dependence on machines or medication, especially when this means existence in an irreversible vegetative state which can last hours, days, months, or years and even decades, an existence assured by pharmacological techniques of "tranquilization."

4. Palliative medicine, so very helpful, has made great progress and should be applied to the fullest extent. Pain therapy can render the

final stages bearable for many incurably sick patients, but it is not the answer for everyone who wishes to die. Nor can pain be relieved in every case of extreme suffering.

(a) The broad spectrum of means available to modern pain therapy brings only "extensive" pain relief – its effectiveness mostly decreasing with time – unless one deprives the patient of all "wakefulness" ("vigilance") and volition, or even renders the patient unconscious. Pain specialists admit that in thousands of cases pains set in which cannot be treated; hospital staff report similar experiences. Physicians recognize that even today, only 85–90 percent of those dying of cancer can be granted "extensive" pain relief.

(b) The wish to die does not arise only from intolerable pain, however, but also from loss of a personal sense of dignity, purpose in life, or prospects for health improvement. Forty-eight percent of Germans (i.e., some 38 million people) could imagine actively assisted death for themselves in the event of lost independence in functions such as eating, breathing, or visiting the toilet (Forsa Survey, October 2000). And when we hear again and again how doctors, care-givers, and judges decide the fates of mortally sick people while ignoring their explicit wish to die (stated in an advanced medical directives or attested by a spouse), we realize that palliative medicine too can be abused, and that there is indisputably a lacuna in the law.

5. For patients suffering from incurable illnesses or injuries with a hopeless prognosis and for neonates with severe malformations incompatible with life, "curtailment of life" following from relief of suffering is admissible.

The new guideline issued by the Federal Medical Council in 1998 informs physicians who previously believed that all technically possible means can and indeed must be put into practice, that there are ethical limits to the preservation of life, and that people should not be maintained indefinitely in conditions of indignity. Assisted death aiming at death "in dignity" has now become, quite rightly, a doctor's duty along with the requirement for "intensive human care." With patients of sound judgment, the wishes of the appropriately informed patient are to be respected "even when these do not conform to diagnostic and therapeutic measures suggested by medical art." Encouragingly, the constant revision of guidelines by the Federal Medical Council is giving ever more prominence to the "patient's right to self-determination." Indeed, "respect" for that right was expressly required for the first time in the most recent formulation of the "Principles," dating from September 1998.

6. Life-prolonging measures may be interrupted "when they only delay death and when progress of the disease can no longer be arrested."

The aim of the Federal Medical Council's Guideline here is to resist the abuse of undoubtedly beneficial medication and equipment. Such "Guidelines" are thus welcome aids in decision-making which prove that German medicine too is willing to learn in questions of allowing to die and caring for the dying, and that opinions previously so divergent have already been reconciled. However, on some issues, many doctors would have expected more courage in taking responsibility for consequences and in offering constructive solutions. We will discuss this further in the sequel.

7. The presumed wishes of the unconscious or irrational patient, as gleaned from some previous declaration of his, are assigned only "special significance" for the final life-and-death decision, and the doctor is supposed to reassess them on the grounds of "the circumstances taken as a whole." This requirement expresses distrust of the patient and scant respect for his conscience.

Those tens of thousands in Germany who have already made their "patient's last testament" will feel that they are still under the tutelage of the doctor, who has the complete and final say. Although the "Principles" first declare that the will of the rationally competent patient is to be respected, they demand, as a matter beyond dispute: "The doctor should help patients who have declined a necessary treatment to reconsider their decision." Physicians themselves criticize such "help" (how many meanings can be read into that word!) as medical paternalism.

8. Like any other will or testament, a patient's advance medical directives must be respected unconditionally (without prevarication or reinterpretation) and should be legally binding.

In an expert opinion written by the well-known jurist from Zurich, Professor Max Keller, the position is expressed as follows:

> A patient's advance medical directives are both admissible and binding (on the addressee). The doctor may deviate from it only if he can prove that it does not correspond to the actual and present wishes of the patient; a possible or hypothetical estimation of the patient's wishes is to be disregarded vis-à-vis the patient's advance directives. The person making the testament may (in a valid manner) appoint a third party (in the sense of an executor) to make sure that the deposition is duly observed. This appointee can enforce the Patient's Testament; the treating physician cannot appeal to medical confidentiality vis-à-vis the appointee.

A U.S. federal law, (the Patient Self-Determination Act of 1991) obliges health institutions to inform patients of their right to decide themselves about a treatment or its cessation and to record their desire in the matter in writing. In several U.S. states, patients must sign "do not resuscitate" orders" before undergoing a major operation. In German Patient's Testaments, the administration or continuance of life-maintaining procedures may be rejected, as in cases of permanent brain damage, high-risk operations, irreversible onset of death...

9. Perceiving the growing threat of being held captive in a high-tech medical system, many patients find intolerable the idea of assigning to the doctor alone the final arbitration over their life or death. This erodes the principle of the patient's personal responsibility and is also seen as presumptuous by a growing number of doctors.

Deep down, doctors and judges must feel relieved when they can ultimately pass the decision to the patient or to the responsible next-of-kin. A very recent verdict by the Federal Court (the Kempten Verdict) is a milestone in this regard. It was given in the case of a woman who had been in a coma for three years. The new verdict reversed the conviction of the doctor and the son for discontinuing artificial feeding. Why? The convicting Regional Court had allegedly ignored the wishes of the patient, who, eight years before her death, had expressed her desire for treatment to be stopped under certain circumstances; the chastened Regional Court subsequently handed down an acquittal. From the testimony of several friends and relations of the patient, it transpired that her "fundamental attitude" was that "she did not want to vegetate or waste away, to hang on tubing or to be totally dependent on the help of others." However, this Federal Court decision seems to have made little difference in judicial practice. Only the Oberhausen District Court, on one single occasion, has permitted the interruption of artificial feeding.

10. Welcome progress in hygiene and medicine has granted innumerable people an additional span of life. This has not been realized "naturally" but is, rather, the outcome of human efforts of a highly technical nature. (Life expectancy in Germany, about thirty-five one hundred years ago, is now over seventy!) Yet for many people this development may lead to years of vegetative wasting away (PVS, or permanent vegetative state).

In view of this new situation, the Federal Medical Council has simply taken cover behind the present penal code, declaring dogmatically that the understanding by many doctors of their task, namely positive assistance for people to die with dignity, is "contrary to the medical ethos." A very moderate alternative bill on assisted death, drafted by leading German jurists (J. Baumann, A. Eser, H.G. Koch, M. von Lutterotti, C. Roxin, H.-L. Schreiber, and others), has been in existence since 1986. The proposed text for Paragraph 216, Section 2 runs as follows: "The Court can...refrain from punishment when the homicide serves to end a most severe state of suffering for the patient, a state no longer bearable, that cannot be eliminated or alleviated by other means."

In German law as it stands, the physician is not guilty if he merely puts the lethal dose on the table, but the same physician is subject to severe penalty if he presents this dose to the patient's lips or administers a lethal infusion or injection. This is manifestly a contradiction in the current law and cries out for urgent correction. It is the legislator's task to undertake an adaptation of the law to the conditions of a new epoch.

11. That every doctor will always act in the interest of the mortally sick and assist humanely at their death is unfortunately an assumption belied by experience.

Those who polemicize against the new Law on Assisted Death in the Netherlands hope in private for a "merciful doctor" to attend them when their time comes. But how and where is the average patient to find "the right doctor"? Many a doctor still lacks the necessary sensitivity to questions of the day about dying. Here is just one testimony out of many, a letter I received: "The cases which you have cited [in your book], of comatose old people being returned to life and thus condemned to further wasting away, are no rarity here either. My mother is one of them. Over a hundred years old, she is a human wreck. She gets taken out of bed every day and then sits for hours in her armchair, waiting…. She often talks about dying: 'I think the good Lord has forgotten me.' She has asked the doctor: 'Can't you give me something so that I can die?' I have spoken to the doctor about whether her dose of heart drugs could not be reduced or gradually discontinued, but he simply cannot entertain that idea."

And here is a volunteer in an old-age home: "I soon realized that being able to die [in an old-age home] is in practice very difficult, in contrast to those old people who can spend their last years at home. I often observe how the doctor refers them to hospital, like this lady, well over ninety. She was dying, but in the hospital she was resuscitated by medical techniques and lived on for another four weeks. Could they not have let her fall asleep? There is another old lady, same age, who can only stay in bed, cannot speak or express herself or have any joy. No relations come to visit. Then she contracted pneumonia and had to go to hospital. Since then she only gets tea through a nasal tube." Recently, the sterile gastric tube (PEG) has come into use (about 100,000 patients in 1999, more than half without their permission). For those capable of rehabilitation this is a salvation, but for those about to die it may well mean prolongation of their suffering and demise.

12. Many a doctor would act otherwise toward a doomed patient if there were no fear of investigations by relatives and colleagues, as well as legal sanctions. In view of the current uncertain state of the law, explicit legislative regulation of assisted death is urgently needed, with prevention of its abuse. Current legal practice is becoming ever less appropriate to the realities prevailing in intensive-care units and nursing homes.

(a) For the 900,000 or so people dying annually in Germany, deaths in hospitals, clinics, nursing, and old age homes account for almost 90 percent in some big cities. Is this necessary? Smaller hospitals in particular are interested in high occupancy of their beds, not least for economic reasons. But many doctors now criticize as totally senseless both the medical activism pursued during the very last hours of the dying and their hospitalization. Instead of seeking superfluous transportation to hospital, instead of all the efforts made to order an ambulance or to find a vacant bed and so on, they would prefer to spend time calmly talking with the dying person in preparation for a dignified demise, and time for a prayer.

(b) All respect is due to those doctors who, despite the uncertain state of the law, and at their own risk, adopt this meaningful and humane course of action, preparing the patient for death with a good word and perhaps a paternoster. Without any doubt they help more than all the medical manipulation described and decried in the written depositions we have cited. These doctors deserve the solidarity of the family and the understanding of the courts. They may find themselves justified in the new Federal Court verdict. With the present legal situation, there is hardly a physician today who dares say out loud what he does in secret.

(c) In view of the undisputed gray area, further legal clarification is essential. The homicide Articles 211 and 212 of the Penal Code are not intended for such cases, and Article 216 about killing on demand does not cover all the problems.

13. As an understandable after-effect of the shock from the murderous Nazi policy of enforced euthanasia, extreme sensitivity prevails in Germany about matters linked to assisted death. But self-righteous condemnation of the Netherlands law on assisted death by a few representatives of the Church and politics, and general preoccupation with those dreadful aspects of German history, ignore the reasoning of its proponents and flout the three-quarters of the German population who sympathize with (of course, fully voluntary) "actively" assisted death.

Those who reproach the Netherlands for a "relapse into barbarism" and the like, as if "nothing is sacred there any longer," confirm the prejudice that the German people always goes to extremes: from the euthanasia dictated by the Nazi state to a democracy which deprives the individual of the right to responsibility for his own death. At all events, there is an attempt in Germany to maintain an extreme taboo around the subject. However, the functionaries of Church, state and the professional organizations leading the polemic are actually ignoring the following:

(1) Our population is aware of both the strength of palliative medicine and its limitations and there is a growing groundswell in Germany, as in all developed countries, to give those mortally sick who wish to die the possibility of doing so (67 percent agree that a terminal patient in hospital should have the right to choose death and to demand that the doctor administer a lethal injection. Allensbach, March 2001).

(2) In the United States, so often the forerunner of developments in Europe, the popular vote has already compelled several states to change the law.

(3) In many European countries such as Switzerland, legislation and medical practice are in no way as rigorous as in Germany.

(4) The Netherlands has not, in fact, issued an unconditional *carte blanche* for actively assisted death. The conditions attached are:

the patient's hopeless situation; unbearable suffering; a wish to die expressed repeatedly and arrived at after free and careful reflection; the diagnosis confirmed by a second physician and approval given by a regional committee (a lawyer, a doctor, and an ethicist) with a subsequent report to the state authorities, who check the case. No physician can be compelled to administer assisted death.

14. Passively and actively assisted death cannot be as sharply distinguished in practice as they are in the abstract. The legal distinctions between "direct" and "indirect," "to desire (a consequence)" and "to accept it," "action" and "inaction," become blurred in the gray area of practice.

(a) Anyone condemning the Netherlands must admit in all honesty to a huge ethico-legal gray area in Germany and, in addition, to an irritating moral double-standard. Thus, a few doctors even regard the withdrawal of artificial feeding as "illicit" actively assisted death (and are thus holier than the pope). Yet the Swiss Academy of Medical Sciences considers "passively" assisted death to include not only withholding artificially introduced food and drink from patients in irreversible coma, but also administered oxygen, medication, blood transfusions, and dialysis.

(b) Admittedly, switching off a ventilating machine or an artificial kidney seems to many doctors to be a most "active" form of passiveness (I would say "a contradiction in terms"). This method, recently tolerated even by the Church, has, with some justification, been called "indirect actively assisted death" in legal parlance. Now why should starving or dehydrating a patient to death be permitted as allegedly passively assisted death, while an overdose of morphine is criminal? A slightly larger dose of morphine for gradual onset of sleep would in this case be more merciful and somewhat "more passive" And it is exactly this that innumerable doctors are doing secretly today.

(c) We hear from the medical profession that in Germany, "actively" assisted death is performed daily out of pure compassion. For declared "passively" assisted death too, the consequences are almost always premeditated – but no one is supposed to talk about that. In public, there is vehement opposition to any "actively" assisted death, but in private, the patient is helped to die (and not merely helped while dying). Who is to find out, for example, whether a doctor has given morphine purely to ease pain, even when he is sure that the patient will die sooner as a result (not culpable), or whether he has given the same dose with the intention of inducing the patient's death (culpable)? Indeed many a doctor would avail himself personally of such "actively" assisted death (among colleagues) and may even assist himself to die. But is *Medicus patiens* more privileged than *Homo patiens*? In the hospice movement there is also a considerable body of opinion in favor of a more honest appraisal of actively assisted death, now that the problems around it are no longer taboo. In the United States, growing tolerance has led to new cooperation between the hospice movement and organizations involved with assisted death.

15. It is true that many a wish to die represents first and foremost a desire for human company, closeness, and attention. Nevertheless it is wrong and even presumptuous to disqualify every death wish as *a priori* a pretext. In the Medical Professional Code for German doctors, the Hippocratic Oath, totally out of date in many parts (e.g., doctors' fees), has rightly been replaced with an oath recommended by the World Medical Union that no longer makes mention of "the administration of lethal potions."

We ought to abandon the spurious argument that there is no such thing as a genuine wish to die. Such a wish indeed exists, more often than admitted by doctors or clergymen who are "ideologically" (religiously?) programmed not even to entertain such an idea. For example, an eighty-year-old woman, suffering for almost twenty years from most severe osteoporosis and enduring constant and extreme pain, writes that the wish for a quick death has been her constant companion for seventeen years, but that there is no one to help her. Aware of artificial life maintenance, many people fear a dementia lasting years or total senility.

16. No one should be urged to die, yet no one should be compelled

to live. The decision – made out of conscience, not arbitrarily – must be left to the suffering person (or his legal representative or, possibly, a lawyer). It is presumptuous for an outsider, even a doctor, to judge whether the sufferer is being subjective in feeling that his condition is unbearable. This claim to "autonomy" on the part of the doctor gradually erodes the relationship of trust between physician and patient.

We need clear legislative regulation, so that abuses such as manipulation by the family, social or even economic pressures can be excluded to a maximum, possibly more effectively than in the Netherlands. Abuses can never be completely prevented in any system, just as social pressure arising from increasing excessive age in our population affects every legal system. A patient's economic considerations should never be the decisive factor, but they should not be disparaged from the outset as immoral. The oft-cited relationship of trust between doctor and patient is not endangered by clearly legislated assisted death (as proved by the Netherlands), but it is endangered by the possibility, inherent in the current situation, of the physician's arbitrary disposition over my life, suffering, and death.

17. The Commandment "Thou shall not kill" is more precisely rendered as: "Thou shall not murder" (Exodus 20:13).

(1) Ending a life is murder when, and only when, it stems from base motives, malice, and violence, against the victim's will.

(2) Ending a life is irresponsible when the motives, though not base, are superficial and ill-considered (as when a man in his prime takes his own life because of a career fiasco, without considering his wife and children).

(3) Yet the ending of a life can also be responsible when happening in its due time.

Both the Bible and traditional Catholic concepts hold that "Life is, of possessions, not the highest" (Schiller). The idea that life is beyond our power of disposal is by no means unconditionally valid: risking life for the sake of a higher good, individual and collective defense unto the death of the aggressor, the fatal shot which saves lives when hostages are being taken, and deploying troops at the risk of their lives – all these are regarded as morally acceptable.

18. A person who believes in an eternal life in God need not be concerned about extending earthly life for as "eternally" as possible.

"To everything there is a season, and a time to every purpose under the heaven:

a time to be born and a time to die" (Eccles. 3:1 ff.) – when, finally, hope for a further dignified human life is no more.

After all our experience of the Vatican since the Encyclical *Humanae vitae* (1968), with its total rejection of birth control, we will not be greatly impressed by rash scholastic invocations of the "breach of an ethical dam" or "opening of the sluice gates" that accompany rejection of new legislation. Those who have proclaimed their epochal error on the beginnings of human life in the matter of "artificial" birth control (the pill!) (and have not yet corrected it) should take care when they now arrogate to themselves the claim for sole truth about the end of human life in the matter of "artificially" assisted death. Thus the danger exists that their own Church's moral authority, which is important also to critics of the Church, will fall into yet greater disrepute. However, just as certain doctors are silent for fear of their professional body and its sanctions, so are many Catholic moral theologians, for fear of the the precise technical term for this institution is: the Congregation for the Doctrine of the Faith (Latin: Congregatio pro Doctrina Fidei) and its procedures for disqualifying teachers.

19. Instead of directly or indirectly promoting extreme positions, the Churches should seek mediation between the extremes. In both the Evangelical and Catholic Church, more voices – especially medical and pastoral voices – should be expressing a reasonable middle course on contentious moral questions, and opposition to unfulfillable and inhuman maximalist demands – the irresponsible libertinism of the postmodern mood of freedom ("the unlimited right to suicide") and, at the same time, the equally irresponsible merciless rigorism based

on reactionary defensiveness ("bear the unbearable as given by God, giving yourself unto God!").

To the dismay also of many Evangelical pastors and laypeople, some leaders of the German Evangelical Church are accepting, without sufficiently discriminating, the strict principles of Catholic teaching ("creeping romanization of the Evangelical Church"). No wonder that millions of people, in our republic too, are looking for religious and ethical guidance outside the major churches on questions that range from birth control to assisted death. The leaders of both churches are complaining about the increasing omission of Christian symbols and wording from death notices and about the growing number of anonymous funerals in past years: these phenomena too are related to the loss of credibility by the churches and their leadership.

20. When the termination of life happens in a responsible manner, let there be no mention of "murder" or even of "homicide" or "purposed killing," but rather of "assistance to die," of assistance given, in an inevitable process of dying, out of compassion and regard for the free will of the sufferer. The patient will be said to have "surrendered his life," which, when the time has come to die and the person has been properly prepared, will happen with composure and humility, in diffident gratitude and hopeful expectation, as redelivery of life into the hands of the Creator. He is a God of compassion, not a cruel despot desirous of seeing any human exist to his last in a hell of pain or in sheer helplessness.

Once their time has come and they have been well prepared, more and more people today would like to pass away consciously. They wish for a dignified leave-taking, in an atmosphere, not of dreary hopelessness, but of spiritual comfort, accompanied to the end by doctors and caring staff, relations, and friends, with the hope of perhaps another life in a new Divine dimension, beyond time and space.

Terminal Care of Children

Walter H. Hitzig

P EOPLE TODAY feel a child's dying and death to be something remote, unfamiliar, and frightening. Yet this problem, which we ignore, repress, or face helplessly, is one with which every doctor working in a children's hospital must contend. Reactions to it have changed enormously in the course of time. Today's understanding must likewise be seen in perspective, for it is very subjective and emotionally charged.

Resting on the realm of Christian/Western ideas, the present chapter may seem out of place in a book on Jewish ethics and assisted death. However, both deeper contemplation of this topic and practical experience have shown that religious and denominational differences lose some significance when universally human issues are at stake. Attending at the deathbed of children or parents of Christian, Jewish, Muslim, and Buddhist persuasion, we are always faced with similar ultimate questions; that the answers differ appears to be less significant. It is remarkable that several parents who lost children still send greetings decades later, whereas patients who were cured are at most heard of again only by chance. The shared coping with suffering and death arouses gratitude.

ATTITUDES TO SICKNESS AND DEATH DOWN THE AGES

The perception of sickness and death has undergone frequent changes in the course of more than two millennia. On this topic and on the history of childhood, Philippe Ariès has written fundamental studies [1, 2], the following observations from which are significant for our subject.

In ancient Rome every deceased – even every slave – received a burial place (*loculus*), which often carried an inscription. A gravestone would also be set up for a deceased child, who would be depicted on it together with, and clearly distinguishable from, the adults, his grieving parents.

From the fifth century onwards, these monuments disappear. The early Christians handed their dead over to the church, which interred them *ad sanctos*, that is, near a saint or a martyr, in anonymous mass graves. In the early Middle Ages, starting around the seventh century, portrayals appear on these graves of a joyous collective resurrection of all the saints, meaning all believing Christians. Personal qualities, merits or offenses were of no import at that time.

From the thirteenth to the fifteenth century, the Last Judgment is represented as the end of individual life: the Archangel Michael, under the supervision of Christ the Supreme Judge, weighs up the soul, whose *liber vitae*, hanging about its neck, is its life's final accounting. The Devil is trying to pull one scale pan down to himself, while the supplications of Mary and John are having their effect on the other. This growing personalization finds its eighteenth-century expression in the gravestone art so familiar to us from baroque memorials.

Graves were originally dispersed over open land, but in the course of the centuries they were included in the residential areas of the growing towns. From 1763, enlightened intellectuals in France called for the removal of cemeteries from the towns on grounds of hygiene. The Cimetière des Innocents in Paris was abolished under Louis XVI in 1785–87. Corpses, skeletons, fabrics, and burial offerings were exhumed from ten feet deep and transported in more than a thousand wagonloads to old stone quarries. After a pause during the Revolution, this development was continued into the nineteenth century, when the slogan was: "No cemetery in a town!" Along with the opening of the great boulevards, Haussmann had planned to construct a necropolis seven miles outside Paris, but this could not be realized because of popular opposition. Now (1880) people wanted to live with the dead: "No town without cemeteries!" The same attitude persists to this day. The graves of departed relatives, carefully tended, are visited frequently, in particular on All Souls' Day.

In the country this did not happen: "The little graveyard nestling round the snow-white church, always spruce despite its age, had never been enlarged. Its earth consists literally of the decomposed mortal remains of past generations; to a depth of ten feet there cannot be a grain which has not made its journey through a human organism which once helped dig up the remaining soil" [3]. This description fits our mountain villages to this very day.

The experience of death has likewise undergone great changes: "Death [in the eighteenth century] was also a public ceremony.... It was important that parents, friends, and neighbors be present. Children were brought in: there is no description of a domestic death without some children.... Just consider the care with which the whole sphere of death is kept away from children today" [1, p. 24]. Gottfried Keller recalls [3]:

> Around that time [he was then fifteen] my grandmother fell ill...and after a few weeks we could see that she was going to die..., When she actually reached that stage, which took several days, this duty [of being with her] became a serious and strict exercise.... Custom required the constant presence of at least three people in the room, who were alternately to pray, to pay respects to unfamiliar visitors constantly coming in, and to report to them.... I, who had nothing particular to do and could read fluently, was therefore welcome to them and was kept at the bedside for most of the day.... The men...declared that my grandmother's death ought to make a deep impression on me – one which would always be useful for me.

In that world, a person would feel his death approaching, talk about it, take leave from his surroundings, and seek to "set his house in order" [4].

A profound change gradually set in during the nineteenth century: death was not to be talked about. The dying avoided mentioning it out of consideration for their kin, and they did not even entertain an idea so outrageous. Thus Leo Tolstoy allows the successful merchant Ivan Ilyich to die alone in wordless surroundings until at last he turns in silence to the wall [5]. The subject has been made taboo. Some speculate that death has replaced the former taboo on sex, which has quite disappeared today, and this idea has given rise to the idea of the "pornography of death" [6]. People may no longer speak about the natural causes for the death of a relative or friend, yet every day "consume" death, possibly in the most gruesome of forms, in crime novels and on television. Today this is further reinforced by films, videos, and computer games. Gorer has compared this behavior to the enjoyment of lewd jokes by a highly prudish Victorian society [6].

As an element in this trend, the act of dying is now considered too offensive to be tolerated at home, and those at its threshold are hastily brought to the hospital. There the doctors, under the pressure of unrealistic expectations, perform unnecessary examinations and treatments. It is not by chance that the author of the critical book *The Nemesis of Medicine* chose the pen-name Ivan Illich [7]. Along with talk of mortality and death, mourning by the bereaved has likewise become socially intolerable. The "tamed death" of the Middle Ages has, via the "wild death" of the eighteenth century, become the "forbidden death" of today [8].

These negative or sarcastic judgments were not without foundation until the middle of the twentieth century. However, the sorry state of affairs they censured were noted by the people directly involved, above all by increasingly concerned doctors, because the loneliness of many dying patients in the hospitals had become evident. Since then, opposing movements have occurred in those quarters, with the aim of returning the patient, the object of our technological medicine, to the center of the stage. We will have more to report about this later.

THE CHILD'S PLACE IN SOCIETY

As we have mentioned, the attitude toward children in the Middle Ages was quite indifferent. This has been ascribed to the high infant mortality, which inhibited people from forming emotional attachmentes to very young children. Thus Montaigne: "I have lost two or three [!] children of infant age, not, indeed, without regret, but yet without being much upset" [2]. As late as the seventeenth century, *Le Caquet de l'Accouchée* has a neighbor comforting a worried post-labor woman, the mother of five "little villains": "before they get as far as giving you a lot of worry you will have lost half of them, or even the lot." "The appearance of the child in the family…was too brief and insignificant for it to become engraved in the memory and to demand special attention." In a similar vein, Gotthelf's peasants say about the death of a child, "It's only a kid"; and he reports of the mother of a large number of children: "Every time they bury a child Lisbeth complains that if there were justice in the world, some of hers ought to die too, but none of them ever perishes." In Dante's *Divine Comedy*, unbaptized departed children appear only as inhabitants of the relatively comfortable Limbo [9]. A child who survived the first critical years mingled with the adults and participated in all their activities, as we can see in many old pictures. In the scheme for human aging, "*puer, adolescens, juves, senis*," the term for infancy is absent.

In the eighteenth century "people derived enjoyment from a child as from a pet, an uncivilized little monkey. When it died, as often happened, one or two people were perhaps a but saddened, but as a rule nobody was very bothered: another child would soon be taking its place and it never managed to emerge from a certain anonymity." [2]. This "affection for a pet" was now criticized and rejected by enlightened moralists and pedagogues, who castigated it as unseemly behavior. Their caution against wrongly understood affection for children was an element in their standards of upbringing: all "mollycoddling of children" was to be avoided because, as taught by the doctrine of Original Sin, the human being is wicked by nature. It was now all but inevitable that children would be strictly, often cruelly disciplined and punished [10]. As a result, corporal punishment came to be seen as an essential measure in bringing up children, as proved by innumerable testimonies. For example: "So long as the Golden Age has not arrived, small boys have to be spanked; I still appreciate in retrospect the double kindness of a real round of beating, which, like a storm, released me from an oppressive sultriness and made more room for fresh good behavior." Compare this to the fate of Meretlein in the same book, that extraordinary child who was entrusted to the vicar for "taming" and driven to death by his strictness [3]. How different from today's view that corporal punishment is not only pedagogically mistaken but liable for prosecution!

In the nineteenth century, "the family begins to revolve around the child, which is granted so much significance that it emerges from anonymity. A child can no longer be lost and replaced without great grief; no longer can the process of bringing it up be repeated so frequently.... Later development leads to polarization of social life into the family sphere, on the one hand, and the professional sphere, on the other, and...to the disappearance of the old social structure" [2]. The statistical decline of infant mortality from more than two hundred per thousand newborns in 1875 to less than five per thousand in 1990 [11] reflects the change in attitude toward the value of every child's life.

The small family unit of today, with its only child and relatively older parents, both of them professionally ambitious, has given rise to the "super-mother". Intellectual women, in particular, look after and protect their only child day and night, take it by car to courses and to special lessons in sports, music, ballet, handicraftss and so on, always at the child's demand and always worried about preparing it for its important tasks in the future. Thus they often experience conflict between their personal professional goals and their bad conscience about possibly neglecting their child [12].

NURSING OF SICK CHILDREN

Until well into the nineteenth century, child care was women's domain – mother, midwife, wet-nurse, or godmother. Sick children were nursed at home and often treated by charlatans; academic medicine was concerned with the "bigger" illnesses of adults. A child that had to be hospitalized would usually be assigned to a women's department with female patients of all ages.

> The children's hospital usually evolved from orphanages or foundling homes…[in which] mortality was enormously high; as late as the end of the nineteenth century this reached close to 100 percent in institutions which took in motherless babies…. In the Spedale di S. Maria della Scala in Siena, the former foundling home, one can see at the entrance a fresco by Lorenzo Vecchietta depicting a ladder on which the *esposti*, i.e., the foundlings, ascend to heaven to the Madonna…. In Paris, foundlings were brought to the Hospice des Enfants-Assistés, the place to which, in the mid-eighteenth century, J.-J. Rousseau brought each of his five children in turn, never to see them again. [13]

In no way, however, should the foundling home be equated with an orphanage of the eighteenth century. In these demonstrably magnificent institutions, for example the Waisenhaus auf der Kornamtswiese, opened in Zürich in 1771, half- and full orphans from impoverished lower-middle-class families were given care and sustenance, and brought up in a strict and orderly regime to become good citizens. "There were no exact guidelines as to age. As a rule the orphanage *was to be spared the presence of excessively young children until they had reached one or two years of age*" [14].

For doctors, a sick child was of little interest and indeed a nuisance. At the world's first children's hospital, the Hôpital des Enfants Malades, founded in Paris in 1802, children could be admitted only from the ages of two to fifteen, because the above-mentioned infant mortality in the foundling homes effectively forbade the separation of babies from their mothers. Most children were admitted for reasons of social welfare and thus came from the poorest strata of the population. This social welfare indication for admission was still to be found into the twentieth century [13], but since the middle of twentieth century, the enormous increase in hospital costs has necessitated other solutions.

From the end of the nineteenth century, individual physicians began to examine sick children by the methods that had by then been developed. Thus, exact measurements (such as the child's size, weight, and liquid intake) and chemical analyses of milk and other foods drew attention to the rational and sound nourishment of Infants and children. Discoveries in microbiology and immunology led to an understanding of the infectious diseases so often catastrophic in childhood. Principles of hygiene often proved effective in preventing them. In the course of the twentieth century, vaccinations, vitamins, antibiotics, and so on, when correctly applied, led not only to a drastic decline in infant mortality but to improved health, as seen in the disappearance of rickets and in the faster growth of children, the so-called secular acceleration. All this considerably improved the long-term life expectancy of newborns.

The application of new physiological insights and techniques of medical intensive care to newborns and premature babies has given rise to a new specialization, neonatology. The care of these children has, however, raised new ethical questions in the area between medical progress and patient welfare, particularly when we consider the huge possibilities of intensive medicine [15–17]. The Neonatology Clinic of the University of Zurich has pioneered practical work in this regard [18–20] by holding regular consultations between all the care-giving participants, together with a pastoral worker and under the direction of an ethicist, and has proposed reasonable guidelines [21]. A polemic on this score emanating from certain German pediatric clinics [22, 23] is presumably based more on misunderstanding than on substantial differences. In my opinion, a significant advantage of the "Zurich Model" is the inclusion of nonmedical experts.

When cases of childhood death are being assessed, the current rather confused public debate about "death with dignity" often assumes a special dimension that is usually not considered. The problem lies in the definition, assumed for adults, of dignity as a social attribute. More precisely we should think of contingent dignity as an acquired status in a task of self-fashioning imposed on people during their lives, a status that may be lost owing to external events. In contrast to this, each and every human being, irrespective of any personal merit, deserves an inherent dignity that is theirs by nature and cannot be ignored [24]. It follows that a newborn child also possesses this inviolate dignity.

Speaking historically, we can see that many people nowadays fear dying but not death. The opposite held true in the Middle Ages, when death entailed punishment and retribution, whereas the natural process of dying was accepted as a brief sickness.

ISOLATION OF THE SICK

The success story of pediatrics had some undesirable consequences for children. New knowledge about hygiene showed that the spread of infectious diseases could be stemmed by isolating the patients. Quarantine, a practice successfully prescribed in port cities for the crews of ships arriving from the tropics, made its debut in the new children's hospitals in 1900. This innovation made it possible to largely contain epidemics of measles, chickenpox, and other childhood diseases.

However, during this critical time, patients found themselves more or less in solitary confinement, because until about 1960, house rules required the isolation of sick children, who thus had to be separated from their mothers on admission. Visits from siblings or friends were not permitted. Parents were allowed to visit for only one hour, on Sunday mornings and Wednesday afternoons. The moment that hour ended, the head nurse's bell would clang through all the wards and rooms, in the same way that closing times are announced in museums. All visitors had forthwith to leave the hospital, which resounded for at least for an hour with weeping and lament.

Today we adduce psychological arguments against such strictness. But we should not forget that it was then the norm, with visiting hours very limited in all hospitals. Education too depended on set principles which were strictly applied. As an extreme example of a notorious *furor paedagogicus* from Switzerland in the nineteenth and early twentieth centuries, we might cite the "Children of the Road" project, which was continued for decades. According to its guiding doctrine, gypsies were brutally deprived of their children in order to bring them up "properly." Another murky chapter in Swiss history includes the "children for hire." Until into the twentieth century, orphans and children of poor families were presented at "child auctions," "auctioned off," and then exploited as cheap labor [25, 26].

Rather than shake our heads in disapproval at the strict education and rigid hospital visiting hours in those times, we should be asking ourselves which present-day doctrines might be similarly reproached in fifty or a hundred years' time. All extreme ideas are bound to be short-lived.

INCURABLE DISEASES IN CHILDREN

In the first half of the twentieth century, there was a gradual, persistent change in the reasons for hospitalizing children. The infectious childhood diseases that had once been so commonplace were now seen less often. Children no longer suffered from some of them. Diphtheria, for example, was rendered rare by protective vaccination. For other diseases, out-patient treatment was applicable, as in the case of scarlet fever with penicillin, or else treatment was possible at home, given the smaller families. Pediatricians now turned their attention to diseases previously neglected because regarded as incurable. Thus, congenital malformations, inherited metabolic disorders, and acquired malignant diseases (cancer) have been studied extensively during the past fifty to eighty years.

In the following discussion, we will take the treatment of malignancies, and especially leukemia, as a representative example. Our main observations will apply, *mutatis mutandis,* to other life-threatening sickness, such as heart disease, cystic fibrosis, endocrine disorders, and defects of the immune system.

For the physician, the scientific problems associated with these disorders came first, while the psychological handling of these children, often very sick, and their parents remained largely the task of the caregiver. The doctor's manifest nonacceptance of the death of an adult patient is possibly even more pronounced among pediatricians, because a child ought to have a full life ahead of him. Many doctors, particularly younger ones, understandably experience the death of a patient as a failure of medical art and even as a personal defeat. A ward with such a case would often be avoided during rounds or visited only very briefly. Should a patient die, the doctors were absolved and the nurses took over all the necessary arrangements and responsibilities.

TREATMENT OF ACUTE LEUKEMIA

Toward the end of the 1950s, this passivity on the part of doctors came under increasing criticism in the large clinics [27, 28]. At the Children's Hospital in Zurich in the 1960s, we began to get more deeply involved in the psychological care of leukemic children [29]. This "blood cancer" is actually not frequent in childhood, but everyone involved experiences the sickness as a dramatic incursion into the carefree existence of a child and its happy family life, and thus regard it as a catastrophe. As such leukemia is felt to be more tragic than the continual suffering of a child who is ill from birth.

At the opening of the twentieth century, patients with the acute form of leukemia would die three to four weeks after diagnosis. Survival (or suffering) was prolonged for a few months by giving blood transfusions and, later, by means of antibiotics. New substances with direct action on cell division (cytostatics) signified a turning point (methotrexate in 1948; purinethol in 1952). Many patients suffered relapses after considerably longer survival and finally died, but individual children remained clear of symptoms [30, 31], and some of them are still alive today. These sparks of hope encouraged pediatric hematologists to look for new therapies and to cooperate closely with pharmacologists in order to develop and apply more effective new drugs. This decade-long battle has had considerable success, and the rate of cure for certain forms of leukemia has risen to near 90 percent [32]. Acute childhood leukemia has become a treatable sickness which can often be cured.

PSYCHOLOGICAL CARE OF TERMINAL PATIENTS

Relaxation of Isolation in the 1960s
The treatment of leukemia was demanding and required full cooperation of patients and parents.

ON THE SITUATION OF THE PATIENT:

The first and immediate problem of the leukemic child patient lies in what is probably his first lengthy separation from his mother, as necessitated by hospitalization; it is thus one of the general problems that arise from the hospitalization of a child [13, 33]. Early childhood, the age most prone to acute leukemia, is undoubtedly a most unsuitable phase for the separation of a child from its parental home.... Most children then have to realize that the power of their parents is limited.... The child feels betrayed and abandoned by its parents and gets into a state of panic or despair.... ost children soon give up resisting, become apathetic, and let anything be done to them; in the ward they are praised as "good children." Frequently the suppressed aggression is turned against the parents so that their first visits can be very dramatic, and, for the mothers, very disappointing.

ON CARE FOR PARENTS AND RELATIONS:

As soon as the diagnosis has been confirmed, we require a personal discussion...which should not be held by telephone.... The doctors must allow themselves ample time to explain clearly and comprehensibly to the parents the diagnosis and possible therapies, the expected course and final prognosis, and also to answer questions.... The meeting should be led by an senior doctor, an expert in the field, but the intern actually treating should always be present and involved, as should an appropriate caregiver.

If you exclude the above two paragraphs, the last sentence above and the following below do not fit together. My suggestion: exclude one sentence before (adjusting the citation number).

The direct disclosure of the diagnosis often seemed to us and others to be almost brutal. A former intern who later specialized in child psychiatry recently admitted to me (forty years later) how appalled he had been by it. Wolf W. Zuelzer, one of the pioneers of pediatric hematology and one of my revered mentors, considered a conversation as delicate as this to be impossible in the presence of others (a doctor, a nurse) but changed his opinion after personal participation. We can state from experience that most parents accepted the discussion as one of honest clarification; many had come to it with the premonition of an extraordinary threat, which was now confirmed. Of course this first conversation was always the beginning of a dialog which was repeatedly resumed in the subsequent period, and was usually taken up with appreciation.

I also emphasized that "the patient should, if possible, be treated throughout by the same doctor." This demand was difficult to realize even in 1965 [29] and has become even more problematic in today's clinics. I felt as well that "The clinic must keep the family doctor fully informed and involve him in the subsequent treatment." Finally,

> *Principles of therapy:*
> A well-known sequence of therapeutic steps is introduced during recovery. The therapeutic measures are initially very intensive, then become considerably milder but remain necessary for a long period in order to prevent relapse. In the event of a relapse, the plan must be reconsidered.

This concept is still valid today. Therapy has become more varied and intensive [32]. As always we first strive to attain a total cure. However, even when the course of events is unfavorable, the physician will not be inactive but will apply every available means to alleviate suffering, the aim now becoming palliative. Today, doctors in such situations can avail themselves of guidelines [17] that will help them make decisions.

PATIENT AUTONOMY SINCE THE 1970S

All these efforts were logical and procedurally correct, since their goal was optimal medical provision for the patient. From today's perspective, however, they did not give sufficient value to the perspective of the patient. Again we must take into account the state of ideas prevalent at the time. For the first time in medical history, doctors disposed of powerful and efficient agents against fatal diseases, and any objection to using these agents was almost unthinkable. It was only with experience that they began to recognize the new burdens being imposed on the patient. Side-effects that led to new, hitherto-unknown complaints or to permanent defects, uncertainty lasting for years coupled to permanent fear of relapse – these demanded totally new attitudes from those affected. These problems have been discussed at various levels since the 1960s.

FRANK DISCOURSE WITH THE PATIENT

"Interviews with the Dying"

In simple conversations with mortally sick people, the psychiatrist Elisabeth Kübler-Ross began to address directly the topic of dying, which had until now been avoided [34]. The doctors at the clinic were extremely skeptical about her aims and only in rare cases allowed her access to "their" patients. Mrs. Kübler found that most of her very sick patients had a clear insight into their inevitable fate. Till then they had been left in lonely isolation because no one was willing to talk about their overriding concern, when, in fact, they themselves had a sound premonition of what lay ahead, even without medical confirmation. They found release in a conversation, previously taboo, about their approaching end.

Mrs. Kübler discerned five phases in this growth of inner awareness:

1. A desire not to admit reality and consequent isolation: the bitter truth is unbelievable and the subject seeks to ignore it by sealing himself off from his surroundings.
2. Anger: reality has overtaken the patient and he rails against his fate: "Why me?"

3. Second thoughts: perhaps the unfavorable outcome can still be avoided.
4. Depression.
5. Assent and tranquility.

Kübler-Ross showed that guidance through the phases of this process is a significant task for the doctor. The moods of the progression she describes are expressed in the Book of Ben-Sirach (Ecclesiasticus), chapter 41 [35]. Johannes Brahms set Luther's text to music in the third of the *Ernste Gesänge*.

1. O death, how bitter are you, when remembered by a man who enjoys good days and plenty and lives without a care,
2. and who is well in all things and can still eat well!
3. O death, how good are you to the needy,
4. who is weak out there and old, all stuck in worries and with nothing better to hope for or expect!

Mrs. Kübler's book claimed immediate and widespread attention; it was translated into many languages and appeared in numerous editions. She had sensed a latent trend, proving it with facts and clearly formulating changes in attitude that derive from it. While Mrs. Kübler conducted her interviews with adults, particularly with the elderly, it was obvious to us that her basic findings also applied to the care of mortally sick children and their parents. They too go through these five emotional phases, and conversation with them must enter into their particular condition. Our own discussion, as described above, were thus in part confirmed and justified, but in part had to be significantly modified and made more "humane."

THE SILENT WORLD OF DOCTOR AND PATIENT
In the light of his experience, the internist and jurist Jay Katz has searchingly criticized the doctor-patient relationship and found that the "patient's participation in decision making is an idea alien to the

ethos of medicine." [36]. Doctors could appeal to the Hippocratic Oath:

> One should carry all this out with such calm and skill that during the treatment, the patient hardly notices anything. One should make dispositions with a friendly and cheerful mien for what must happen. Free yourself of your own thoughts, but as to the patient, now reproach him bitterly and with severity, now encourage him with consideration and attentiveness. Let the patient notice nothing of what will happen and what threatens him – for many have been driven by this, I mean by the above prediction of the threatening future and subsequent fate, to extreme acts. [37]

Katz continues that around 1950 a majority of the medical profession rejected giving the patient exact information (cf. [1]). No expert would have dared to testify against a doctor, because a "conspiracy of silence" seems to have prevailed [36, p. 56]. Instead of this, we ought to think again and speak openly with the patient: "The art of conversing with patients has to be painstakingly learned " (p. 78).

In the wake of several lawsuits, courts in the United States began to ask in the late 1950s (p. 59) whether "patients [are] entitled not only *to know what* the doctor proposes to do but also *to decide whether* an intervention is acceptable in light of its risks and benefits and the available alternatives, including that of no treatment?" (p. 59). Patients had always enjoyed legal protection against fraud and deception by doctors, but the new aim was "that the physicians should be placed under an affirmative duty to acquaint patients with the important risks and plausible alternatives to a proposed procedure."

The courts had always respected the authority of the doctors: "The law had always respected the arcane expertise of physicians and rarely held them liable if they practiced good medicine," but this principle was now being questioned in certain cases. Pronouncing judgment in the case of a professional error, Judge Bray of the California Court of Appeals declared on October 22, 1957: "In discussing the element of risk, a certain amount of discretion must be employed consistent with the full disclosure of facts necessary to an informed consent" (p. 61). Thus was coined the catchphrase "informed consent," which, since then, cannot be omitted from any discussion of medical ethics. The British objection that the adjective "informed" is superfluous (Laurence: "consent is consent is consent," after Gertrude Stein [38]) went unheeded. It is axiomatic today that in clinical trials of new medications, the informed consent of the subject must be obtained [39]. Ethicists demand in the same sense that the autonomy of the patient must be fully respected [40].

A devil's advocate might object that this "patient empowerment" has shifted the responsibility for diagnostic and therapeutic decisions in medical practice from the doctor to the patient ("you'll have to decide yourself"), a consideration that may well raise serious new problems. Older patients in particular feel themselves at a disadvantage because they traditionally seek and accept the advice of their physician.

Katz was not primarily concerned with behavior toward the critically ill, but some of his observations were eye-openers to us with regard to conversations with patients and their parents. Our teachers had instilled in us the Hippocratic principle that there is much the doctor must conceal for ethical reasons. We had begun to infringe this principle but without convincing justification. Now we had it: the Hippocratic rules on this question no longer suited the times. A new study of doctors' decisions indicates that there is north–south divide, with the doctor's opinion being more frequently decisive in southern European countries than in the north [41].

DEPTH-PSYCHOLOGICAL ASSISTANCE

In 1968 a visit by Susan Bach to our Children's Hospital in Zurich resulted in a collaboration lasting decades. It has proved to be a blessing for some of our patients and an enrichment for many of our co-workers.

Susan R. Bach was born in Berlin in 1902 [42], where she grew up in a cultured medical household. She concluded her studies in crystallography with a dissertation, but it was not accepted by the university, already dominated by the Nazis. Nonetheless, her background of lucidity in the natural sciences influenced her thinking for life. With other activities denied her, she turned to the care of handicapped children. After briefly attending Carl Jung's lectures in Zurich, she emigrated to England in 1939 with her husband, Hans Bach.

> From 1941 Mrs. Bach worked as a psychotherapist at St. Bernhard's Hospital in London. During her work there, in 1947, she noticed that spontaneously drawn or painted pictures can express the current mental as well as somatic state of the artist. She discussed her idea with Jung, who encouraged her to collect material and continue her research. After a lecture seminar by Mrs. Bach in 1958 at the university's Psychiatric Clinic, both C.A. Meyer, then director of the Jung Institute, and Hugo Krayenbühl, director of the Department of Neurosurgery at the University Hospital, Zurich, evinced interest in scientific collaboration with her. A publication of the initial results aroused the attention of the profession [43].

Access to patients in the Neurosurgical Clinic was made possible by Hans-Peter Weber, at that time a scientific draftsman, who began compiling a prudent and precise collection of patients' drawings. He was not satisfied with merely accumulating pictures but also collected comments by the patients about their work and data from their medical histories. The assessment of this "documentary material" by Susan Bach proved to be an important event. She looked carefully at every detail of a picture, searching for some connection to the physical state of its creator (she called it "organic vision"). Thorough analyses of some cases confirmed her in her conviction that a patient can directly depict a somatic finding (e.g., a brain tumor). She wished to continue her research with other patients, and, at the suggestion of Prof. Krayenbühl, critically sick children provided a new group for her studies.

I met Mrs. Bach in 1970, perhaps with some reservations. Her project did not seem to burden our patients, and it corresponded to my own inclinations. While still a junior doctor, I had run regular "drawing competitions" in the legendary Ward 4 with its twenty-four children, all of whom participated. The works of art were exhibited when the head of department visited. They were seriously appraised and even rewarded with a prize (for every participant!) by Prof. Fanconi. But beyond some enjoyable entertainment for everyone involved, we attached no particular importance to these activities at the time.

I suggested to Mrs. Bach that she examine children with acute leukemia. My skepticism changed dramatically after the first seminars Mrs. Bach held with our hematology group. We found her approach unusual and surprising because she made no pretense of knowing or being able to "explain" everything, unlike some child psychiatrists ("the tree has no earth and no roots; that means…"; "the red expresses aggression…"). Instead, she would contemplate each picture silently and repeatedly. Then she would ask us: "What do you see there?" She tolerated the long and embarrassing initial silence, which lasted until some hesitant and diffident answers emerged, particularly from the youngest members, who normally did not dare to say very much. She encouraged everybody to mention even apparently minor details. To our surprise, the discussion became more lively and relaxed; seemingly random details developed before our eyes into a multifaceted picture. Susan Bach concluded the session in a manner that surprised us again, by inviting us to attempt an overall survey of the present condition of the child. This was a paradigm of "Socratic midwifery."*

PICTURES BY LEUKEMIC CHILDREN

We could see for ourselves that children in the initial acute phase of the disease hardly used colors. That is why we dubbed the scheme the "White Child Project" (in 1847 Virchow had named it leukemia [i.e., "white blood"]). Here is an example: Xaver had been diagnosed at the age of eleven with acute myeloblastic leukemia. On reception he was bleeding massively from the mouth and nose. The picture he drew (see "My Doctor," Fig. 1, no. 49 in [44, 45]) shows a pale figure in a soiled white doctor's coat, with a red bulbous nose and red mouth. On checking we found that the doctor's tunic was completely clean, but the stains in the picture corresponded exactly to the patient's hematomas. The rigidity of the right arm is authentic, because the artist's arm was immobilized for a blood transfusion and the drawing was done with the left. The patient had thus represented his own bodily condition in a lifelike manner. There were lightning flashes over the head of the figure, or perhaps emerging from it. The boy comments: "It knocked off his head" – so that is what he felt like.

We were also impressed by the way the pictures changed under the influence of treatment. Eight-year-old and hitherto healthy Urs entered the department with severe anemia. On his first day in hospital with acute lymphatic leukemia, he too used no colors. A few days later, and after two blood transfusions (hemoglobin up from 49 to 97 g/l), he drew "Red Water" (Fig. 2, no. 6 in [44, 45]): Standing on wavy dark-green ground is a little man, head and body outlined in blue and his belly all filled in with red. He is watering a red flower with red water from a red hose – a moving representation of the feeling of vitality that the blood transfusion has restored to Urs. The huge flower on a pale-green stalk, with eight petals (Urs's age), stands almost as tall as the little figure itself: is this his *arbor vitae*? The golden sun, whose mouth, nose, and eyes are likewise colored red, shines in a friendly way on the world. Urs was in fact cured, and returned to visit us many years later when he was a capable apprentice.

The picture by seven-year-old Marina, "The Red Cowshed" (Fig. 3a, no. 205 in [44, 45]) drew our attention to the hopeless loneliness of this shy little girl. She was brought into the clinic with acute lymphatic leukemia. At first she refused to speak or to eat. During that time she drew a picture of a crooked red house without doors and windows, against bare surroundings (no ground, no sky, no sun); she explained: "This is a cowshed. The cows are mooing because they are hungry. The farmer has gone into the forest and forgotten them. No one is coming." In two short conversation the child psychologist was able to help her out of her isolation. A few days later Marina drew a little man (Fig. 3b, no. 30 in [44, 45]) and explained: "The little man has had a lot to eat and is feeling good. All the birds [seven, drawn in violet] are flying toward the sky, but the smallest will get there first." Marina was the youngest of four children. On the ground there are seven mountain daisies, of which the last one on the left has no flower. The little man's left hand has four long fingers, and the right hand, three, all together seven (pictures are always arranged mirror-image fashion). Seven days later Marina died peacefully, in the seventh year of her life.

According to Susan Bach, one should always pay attention to numbers. We have another example with Lisbeth, a five-year-old rural girl who was admitted with acute lymphatic leukemia. She died almost three years later after a stormy sickness with several remissions and relapses. "The Flower with the Devil's Mask" (Fig. 4, no. 18 in [44, 45]) is the fifth of a row of seven flowers in the large garden of a beautiful half-timbered house. The first four flowers grow out of dark-green leaves, while the green of the last three is pale and weak. Among these fine round blossoms, the fifth one, with a devil's mask, is disturbingly ugly – the disease had started in the child's fifth year, and in her eighth she died. In several other pictures by Lisbeth, Mrs. Bach interpreted numbers that appeared repeatedly in terms of relevant dates in the child's life. We have already pointed out the seemingly significant numbers in the cases of Urs and Marina.

> Many pictures display feelings of fear, apprehension, threats, or scenes of strife. Among the more than three hundred pictures drawn by Adrian we have chosen "Sea Battle" (Fig. 5a, no. 191 in [44, 45]). He was taken ill at the age of six with acute lymphatic leukemia, which could at first be brought into remission. For two years, regular ambulatory check-ups in our clinic excepted, he led a normal and happy life. At the age of eight he had relapses in the bone-marrow and meninges, to which he succumbed a year later despite intensive treatment. Our picture shows dramatic scenes in ten different colors on a large pale-yellow sheet. Two sailing ships seem to be interlocked at the bows. Pirates, identified by the skull-and-crossbones flag on the upper far left, are attacking from the ship on the left. It has a stout mast with a big manned crow's nest and fully billowing sails, while the sails of the ship on the right are slack, tentlike, and hanging from an invisible mast. A violent fight is raging on deck: seven brown-clad pirates with an assortment of stabbing weapons and firearms, are attacking, presumably from

the left, eight (blue-clad) men on the right. Seven cannons are visible in the seven angular gun-ports below deck. Streaks of fire and smoke suggest two shots just fired. The seven gun-ports on the ship under assault are empty (or closed?). Some of the blue sailors have their hair standing on end, there are hats flying in the air, and over one bent (falling?) blue man far on the right there is a large question mark – what is he wondering about? The waves are rigid and angular, like rocks. Much of the hull of the right-hand ship is no longer in contact with the water.

"Viking Ship," too, shows a ship in peril on a stormy sea (Fig. 5b, no. 192 in [44, 45]) . On deck we see ten Vikings of various sizes, colors, and weaponry. All the weapons are raised. But for the ten men there are only nine shields. Six blood-red stripes cover part of the billowing sail; there is room for three more stripes in the space on the right, which has been left white. Up in the spacious crow's nest there is an eleventh man, with a telescope. Six little lines above his head presumably denote his sudden alertness. We know from his case history that Adrian enjoyed six years of full-blooded good health and then sickened with "white blood," that he enjoyed two more years of protection by treatment but then suffered relapses; despite subsequent more intensive treatment, always with the hope of saving him, he succumbed, after a dogged struggle, in his tenth year.

> Many similar cases convinced us that bodily states and their changes in the course of an illness can be displayed in pictures. The seminar sessions with Susan Bach soon became well-known in the whole department and were attended by colleagues from outside the hematology group. In 1977 we organized an open three-day colloquium with several invited guest speakers, which I called "The Bach Festival" [46, 47].

A substantial objection to Mrs. Bach's method was her subjective, intuitive procedure and the method's questionable reproducibility. She was able repeatedly to convince even critical audiences, but people

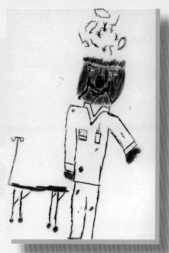

Fig. 1 Xaver, aged 11,
(AML) "My Doctor"

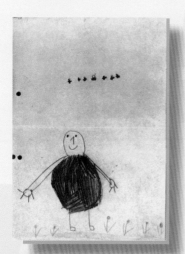

Fig. 3b Marina, aged 7,
(ALL) "All Birds Fly in the Sky"

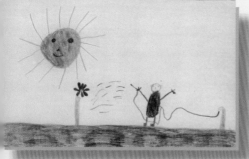

Fig. 2 Urs, aged 8,
(ALL) "Red Water"

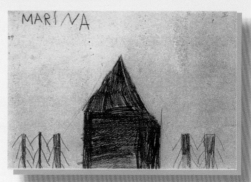

Fig. 3a Marina, aged 7,
(ALL) "The Red Cowshed"

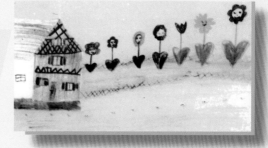

Fig. 4 Lisbeth, aged 8,
(ALL) "The Flower with the Devil's Mask"

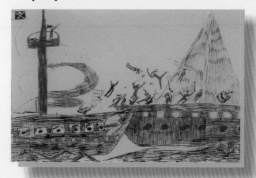

Fig. 5a Adrian, aged 8,
(ALL) "Sea Battle"

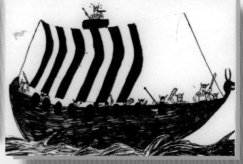

Fig. 5b Adrian, aged 8,
(ALL) "Viking Ship"

AML): acute myoblastic leukemia; **(ALL):** acute lymphatic leukemia

protested that only she was competent in it, and that she had founded no "school." We urged her for years to work on this matter; her previous training in crystallography would provide her with the necessary foundations. She took this criticism seriously and worked for several years on her book. Having been granted a long life, she was able to bring the work to a successful conclusion in 1990 [44], with a German edition in 1995 [45].

Her method, thus scientifically assured, can now be both taught and learned. She establishes clear rules for a systematic examination of pictures, giving it a theoretical and empirical basis. This includes counting entities and their repetition, the arrangement of items in the four quadrants of the picture, the nature and distribution of colors, the use of archetypal themes, and finally the explanation and commentary of the artist. As the sickness takes its course, changes in all these features must also be noted.

THE SUSAN BACH / KASPAR KIEPENHEUER SCHOOL

Even a school of teaching will only remain alive if its devotees pass on the message. Young people from various parts of the world made the effort to acquire the necessary training, almost all of them coming from the field of psychology. They visited Susan Bach in London or studied at the C.J. Jung Institute in Zurich. For them the method was of interest in various areas of psychotherapy. Presumably some of them worked further with it, but we have lost personal touch with them.

One exception was Kaspar Kiepenheuer, a trained medical man and pediatrician. He had been assigned to my Hematology Department in 1970 for the pediatric rotation of his training. The work with mortally sick children was a shock, "made him speechless" as he put it. He performed his scientific and technical tasks satisfactorily but felt insecure and unhappy. For him the acquaintance with Susan Bach proved to be a watershed. With her counsel he devoted himself to the psychological condition of his patients with an intensity unwonted for our clinic, visited them at home after their release, had long evening discussions with their parents, and also showed concern for the siblings, who were often being deprived. He pursued his observation of the process of dying with sympathy. He impressively demonstrated to us that a child, too, in no way dies without awareness, but instead, in the course of a long illness, can foresee death and accept it, so that life's cycle is completed [48, 49]. He portrayed several such fates movingly and in beautiful language, using appropriate pictures as illustrations [49]. After additional training in child psychiatry, he devoted himself entirely to this area. In further publications and case studies he treats other problems (puberty, break with the parental home, etc. [50]), always using the artistic works of the patients as a valuable tool, together with the empathic consideration and judgment that were Susan Bach's. Sadly, Kaspar Kiepenheuer himself succumbed to cancer at a young age, without finding a direct successor to his work in our clinic.

Assessment

In retrospect, we can state that Susan Bach demonstrated a new approach to mental developments in critically sick children and in her book handed down practical guidance in this regard. Her method can thus be learned. Its didactic value for our clinic was inestimable. Among other things, we have learned:

> That ideas about life's end preoccupy even very small children, and can be profoundly intense for adolescents.
>
> That the sense of a life cycle coming to a close can be observed even in children. When they develop this sense, their death no longer seems completely senseless to them. Proper attention and care for the dying child can be very helpful
>
> That the stage of dying is part of every doctor's existence and experience, as much in pediatrics as in any other specialty.
>
> That a physician must reflect on dying and death.
>
> That one can and must speak to patients and/or their parents about dying and death.
>
> That doctors must be taught and must learn this manner of dialogue.

Current Practice in Psychological Support

It is obvious that the intensive depth-psychological care we have described must not be generalized and can be offered only to individual patients. There are various other means that have proved helpful for those in need.

Self-help groups. Many rare diseases can today be treated effectively. Apart from a few specialists, those patients and their families often know more about coping with the disease than other doctors or care-givers. They often establish special-interest groups, and in fact there are now several dozen of these in Switzerland. The group members advise each other, organize joint activities, and often work outside the group, for instance in dealing with insurance companies. Parents of children with cancer have been organized since the 1970s, initially with the help of Susan Bach, and their groups has since achieved a great deal. It keeps hospitalized children occupied with artistic activities (art therapy) and with cheerful entertainment, such as visits by clowns and magicians. The group provides parents with information and support. In conjunction with other such groups, it organizes summer camps in Switzerland in which a patient's parents and siblings can participate, and it raises considerable sums of money for these activities. Thanks to the generous support of a private foundation, a house was built near the clinic in Zurich, where parents and children can stay under favorable terms during courses of treatment. Finally, in cooperation with the cantonal Anti-Cancer League, this group has facilitated effective support for certain research studies in the clinic.

Terminal support givers. Women who have lost a child to the disease often volunteer to advise other parents and children. In preparation for this, they are offered psychological training and counseling.

Psychological support by professional staff. With the help of funds from the Anti-Cancer League and a private foundation, our Children's Clinic has been able to employ two people trained in clinical psychology (1.5 positions) to counsel children and their parents. Here again, there is the danger of possible estrangement between the patient and the doctor.

Summary and Conclusions

Attitudes toward dying and death have changed in many ways, sometimes contradictory, in the course of the centuries. The subject became taboo in the nineteenth and twentieth centuries, and ever higher walls of silence were built around the dying. Critics became concerned about the resulting isolation of dying patients and their next-of-kin, while doctors pointed out the danger of Western society running into a fatal blind alley, to the great detriment of all concerned.

At about the same time, attitudes toward children were changing. Perceived as an anonymous class in the Middle Ages, they became individual and cherished only children. High child mortality, once fatalistically accepted, began to be reduced thanks to social and medical advances. The taboo about death was doubly reinforced, however, and the death of children was suppressed as totally unacceptable.

In addition to their scientific efforts, doctors involved in treating diseases that still have early fatal outcomes are challenged by the task of giving these endangered patients appropriate psychological care and support. First of all, this requires that the doctor understand the limitations of medicine, a difficult demand to make, particularly of young doctors. Only after this inhibition has been overcome is it possible to engage in frank discourse with the sick child and the parents. We were surprised to find that many of those affected already had an inkling of the bitter truth and were glad of any opportunity to talk with trained medical personnel, other troubled parents, or clergy.

The medical care of patients who cannot be cured by current medical means must be supplemented by relief (palliative) measures, not discussed here, and by the provision of psychological support, for which we cite numerous possibilities. These include well-planned discussions, which may be usefully introduced by the children's artistic work, stimulating distractions, particularly in the company of other such patients, treatment by staff trained in psychology, and so on. It is not unusual for parents and care-givers to discover that children are capable of understanding death as the rounding off of a life's course, however brief, and of accepting it as such.

Our preoccupation with this difficult subject has convinced us that answers of lasting validity will never be found to questions such as these about the end of life. Instead, every generation will have to think them through in its own era and find the best course of action consonant with the social trends at that time. But one rule must always be respected: *Salus aegroti suprema lex* ("The patient's welfare is the supreme rule").

Acknowledgments

Reproduction of our patients' pictures [45] was made possible by the kind permission of Daimon Verlag, Einsiedeln (Dr. R. Hinshaw) and the Susan Bach Foundation (Küsnacht). I am grateful to the librarians of the Children's Hospital, the Institute for the History of Medicine, and the Zurich University Hospital for assembling the scientific literature.

Notes

1. P. Ariès, *Studien zur Geschichte des Todes im Abendland*, vol. 1 (Munich and Vienna: Carl Hanser Verlag.1976).
2. P. Ariès, *Geschichte der Kindheit*, vol. 1, 8th ed. (Munich: Deutscher Taschenbuch Verlag, 1988).
3. G. Keller, *Der grüne Heinrich* (Frankfurt a/M: Insel Verlag, 1980).
4. Isaiah 38:1.
5. P. Ariès, "Der Kranke, die Familie und der Arzt," in *Studien zur Geschichte des Todes im Abendland*, ed. P. Ariès (Munich and Vienna: Carl Hanser Verlag, 1976), pp. 190–201.
6. G. Gorer, *Death, Grief and Mourning in Contemporary Britain: A Study of a Contemporary Society* (New York: Doubleday, 1965).
7. I. Illich, *Die Nemesis der Medizin: die Kritik der Medikalisierung des Lebens* (Munich: Beck, 1955).
8. P. Ariès, "Der ins Gegenteil verkehrte Tod. Die Veränderung der Einstellungen zum Tode in den westlichen Gesellschaften," in *Studien zur Geschichte des Todes im Abendland*, ed. P. Ariès (Munich and Vienna: Carl Hanser Verlag, 1976), pp. 157–189.
9. L. Villiger, Personal communication to Dante: *Divina Commedia*.
10. U. Kronauer, "Verhätscheln verboten. Die 'Affenliebe,' im 18. Jahrhundert," *Neue Zürcher Zeitung* 2./3 (August 2003).
11. M. Bopp and F. Gutzwiller, "Die mittlere Lebenserwartung in der Schweiz – historischer und internationaler Hintergrund und einige Gedanken zur zukünftigen Entwicklung," *Soz. Präventivmed.* 43 (1998): 149–161.
12. D. Schoeller Reisch, "Die neuen Übermütter. Rückschau und Fragen zur Genese eines Rollenbildes," *Neue Zürcher Zeitung* 2./3 (August 2003).
13. G. Fanconi, "Die Hospitalisation des Kindes. Séminaire sur l'hospitalisation des enfants," *Helv. Paediatr. Acta.* 18 (1963): 558–568.

14. M. Crespo, "Verwalten und Erziehen. Die Entwicklung des Zürcher Waisenhauses 1637–1837," *Mitteilungen der Antiquarischen Gesellschaft in Zürich*, vol. 68 (Zürich: Chronos Verlag Zürich, 2001).
15. M. Cuttini et al., "End-of-Life Decisions in Neonatal Intensive Care: Physicians' Self-Reported Practices in Seven European Countries: EURONIC Study Group," *Lancet* 355 (2000): 2112–2118.
16. P.J. Sauer, "Ethical Dilemmas in Neonatology: Recommendations of the Ethics Working Group of the CESP (Confederation of European Specialists in Paediatrics)," *European Journal of Pediatrics* 60 (2001): 364–368.
17. W.H. Hitzig and R. Ritz. "Medizinisch-ethische Richtlinien zu Grenzfragen der Intensivmedizin. Directives concernant les problèmes éthiques aux soins intensifs" (http://www. samw.ch).
18. T.M. Berger et al., "Empfehlungen zur Betreuung Frühgeborener an der Grenze der Lebensfähigkeit (Gestationsalter 22–26 ssw)," *SAeZ* 83 (2002): 1589–1595 (http: //www.samw.ch).
19. G. Duc, "Neonatologie et Ethique: chronique d'un conflit annoncé. Conférence donnée le 4.9.200 3à l'occasion des 80 ans du Prof. E. Gautier," *Paediatrica*.14 (2003): 45–50.
20. R. Baumann-Hoelzle, "An der Schwelle zum eigenen Leben," *Dialog Ethik*, vol. 3 (Bern: Peter Lang, 2002).
21. K. von Siebenthal and R. Baumann-Hoelzle, "Ein interdisziplinäres Modell zur Urteilbildung für medizinisch-ethische Fragestellungen in der neonatalen Intensivmedizin," *Ethik Med.* 11 (1999): 233–245.
22. H. Hepp et al., "Grenzen ärztlicher Behandlungspflicht bei schwerstgeschädigten Neugeborenen. Einbecker Empfehlung, revidierte Fassung 1992," *Ethik Med.* 4 (1992): 103–104.
23. V. von Loewenich, "Ethische Probleme bei Frühgeborenen," *Monatsschr. Kinderheilkd.* 151 (2003): 1263–1269.
24. H. Rüegger, *Sterben in Würde? Nachdenken über ein differenziertes Würdeverständnis* (Zürich: NZZ Buchverlag, 2003).
25. J. Gottheit, *Der Bauernspiegel oder Lebensgeschichte des Jeremias Gotthelf* (La Chaux-de-Fonds: F. Zhan, 1837).
26. A. Honegger, *Die Fertigmacher* (Frauenfeld: Huber,1986).
27. J. Bernard and J.M. Alby. "Problèmes psychologiques posés par la leucémie aigue de l'enfant," *Courrier.* 6 (1956): 135.
28. S.B. Friedman et al., "Behavioral Observations on Parents Anticipating the Death of a Child," *Pediatrics* 32 (1963): 610–625.
29. W.H. Hitzig, "Psychologische Probleme bei der Behandlung der Leukämie im Kindesalter. Standpunkt des Klinikers," *Helv. Paediatr. Acta.* 20 (1965): 48–55.
30. J.H. Burchenal, "Long-Term Remissions in Acute Leukemia – Spontaneous or Induced," In *Xth Congr. Int. Soc. Haemat.* (Stockholm, 1964).
31. C. Gasser, "Langdauernde Remissionen akuter Leukämien im Kindesalter," *Med. Klin.* 50 (1964): 385–393.
32. A. Reiter et al., "Intensive ALL-type Therapy without Local Radiotherapy Provides a 90% Event-Free Survival for Children with T-cell Lymphoblastic Lymphoma: A BFM Group Report," *Blood.* 95 (2000): 416–421.
33. A.M. Bongiovanni, "Hospitalization of Children: Report of an International Seminar," *Pediatrics.* 34 (1964): 1–3.

34. E. Kübler-Ross, *On Death and Dying* (New York: Macmillan, 1969).
35. J. Sirach, Apokrypha: 41. Kap. in M. Luther, *Bibel* (Stuttgart: Privileg. Württembergische Bibelanstalt, 1934), p. 64.
36. J. Katz, *The Silent World of Doctor and Patient* (London: Collier Macmillan,1984).
37. R. Kapferer, *Die Werke des Hippokrates. Die hippokratische Schriftensammlung in neuer deutscher Übersetzung* (Stuttgart and Leipzig: Hippokrates-Verlag, 1934).
38. D.R. Laurence, "Informed Consent." *Lancet* 341 (1993): 1479.
39. W.H. Hitzig and W. Baer. "Medizinisch-ethische Richtlinien für Forschungsuntersuchungen am Menschen. Directives médico-éthiques pour la recherche expérimentale sur l'homme," *SAeZ.*78 (1997):1585–1600 (http://www.samw.ch).
40. D. Gill et al., "Guidelines for Informed Consent in Biomedical Research Involving Paediatric Populations as Research Participants," *Eur. J. Pediatr.* 162 (2003): 455–458.
41. A. van der Heide et al., "End-of-Life Decision-Making in Six European Countries: Descriptive Study," *Lancet* 362 (2003): 345–350.
42. R. Goldstein, *Images, Meanings and Connections: Essays in Memory of Susan R. Bach* (Einsiedeln: Daimon Verlag, 1999).
43. S.R. Bach, "Spontanes Malen schwerkranker Patienten," *Acta Psychosomatica* 8 (1966).
44. S.R. Bach, *Life Paints Its Own Span. On the Significance of Spontaneous Paintings by Severely Ill Children*, vol. 1 (Einsiedeln: Daimon Verlag, 1990).
45. S.R. Bach, *Das Leben malt seine eigene Wahrheit. Über die Bedeutung spontaner Malereien schwerkranker Kinder*, vol. 1 (Einsiedeln: Daimon Verlag, 1995).
46. S.R. Bach, "On the Archetypal Motif of the Bird: Pictures of Severely Ill Patients with Parallels from Works of Art to Wall Paintings of Early Man," *Psychosomatic Medicine* 9 (1980).
47. S.R. Bach, "Guidelines for Reading and Evaluating Spontaneous Pictures," *Psychosomatic Medicine* 9 (1980).
48. W.H. Hitzig and K. Kiepenheuer, "Das Kind und der Tod. Gedanken zur Beziehung zwischen Pädiater und todkrankem Kind," *Hexagon Roche* 4 (1976): 1–10.
49. K. Kiepenheuer, "Spontaneous Drawings of a Leukemic Child: An Aid for More Comprehensive Care of Fatally Ill Children and Their Families," *Psychosomatic Medicine* 9 (1980).
50. K. Kiepenheuer, *Geh über die Brücke. Die Suche nach dem eigenen Weg am Beispiel der Pubertät.* (Zürich: Kreuz Verlag, 1988).

The Report of the Public Committee on Matters Concerning the Terminally Ill Patient

DRAFT LAW, REPORT, AND DIVERGENT OPINIONS

The draft law is rendered in full. In order to avoid repetition and excessive length, only the most relevant excerpts from the commission's report are given, including some historical background, discussions, and divergent opinions.

CHAPTER 1: HISTORICAL AND CURRENT BACKGROUND

1. The Dilemmas

The problems involving the patient who is close to death (the "terminally ill patient" or "end-of-life patient") are among the most difficult and controversial questions in modern medicine. They are ethical, medical, social and psychological, religious, halakhic and legal in nature. Dilemmas about the patient close to death affect personally and directly almost every individual, whether in decisions about the end of his own life or that of someone dear to him. The topic is particularly difficult because it involves, literally, fateful life-or-death decisions.

Indeed, the attitude to and care of the terminally ill patient have throughout the ages belonged to the outstanding ethical problems of medical activity. In most of the ancient oaths for physicians, mercy killing by the physician was regarded as a moral transgression (as in the Hippocratic Oath: " I will not give a lethal drug to anyone, even on request, nor will I suggest doing so"). Yet, throughout human history and in all human cultures, diverse schools of thought have encouraged facilitation of death for various sectors of the population, with various justifications. We find examples of this in Stoic attitudes among the Romans and in the behavior of aged Eskimos.

Indeed in recent years, the question of the terminally ill patient has become one of the most acute problems in medical ethics, arousing universal and stormy debate the world over.

Recently, a combination of several causes has exacerbated the moral problems inherent in this subject.

The enormous progress in medical science and technology has led to a significant increase in life-expectancy. Moreover, technological and medical progress now allow us to prolong life in its final stages under conditions and in situations for which this was formerly impossible. Yet herein lies the problem: prolongation of life does not always lead to improved quality of life, and the surviving patients sometimes suffer from severe dysfunction of various organs, physical pain, impaired intellectual function, and severe mental and physical suffering.

There has been an ethical revolution in the doctor-patient relationship, from a paternalism in which the physician decides what is good for the patient and acts accordingly on his own authority, to an autonomistic approach according to which it is the competent patient who decides for himself, within medical, legal, and ethical limits. The patient's deliberate consent is therefore needed for every therapeutic procedure.

Involved in the care of the terminally ill patient are many people with different cultural and philosophical backgrounds, who therefore present a variety of views on what should or should not be done for such a patient.

Today, the general public is much more involved in medico-ethical questions in general, and those affecting the terminally ill patient in particular. This involvement is expressed in, among others, the media, the law, and legislative activity.

In addition, the limited resources for medicine, which cannot grant all possible treatments for all needs, affect the ethical problems related to the terminally ill and sometimes become a consideration in the decision-making process concerning these patients.

The dilemmas surrounding this topic are so manifold and complex that philosophical, legal, and religious justification can be found for almost all directions of theory and practice.

2. The Factual Position in Israel

Today, with the presentation of this report, practical treatment of the terminally ill patient in Israel varies from one medical center, indeed from one department to another, and sometimes from one doctor to the next. The norms applied in Israel regarding terminally ill patients have not been studied and are certainly not uniform.

3. The Legal Position in Israel

Past legislative and legal efforts to solve this dilemma were incomplete and were not applied.

In view of the fact that the problem of the terminally ill patient was not regulated in an acceptable, consistent, and legally binding manner, the then minister of health, Member of Knesset (MK) Rabbi Shlomo Benizri decided to appoint Professor Avraham Steinberg as chairman of a Governmental Public commission charged with formulating a draft bill on the problem of the terminally ill patient. The appointment dated from February 20, 2000. In the interest of thorough and effective debate, the commission was divided into the following four subcommittees, each with its own chairman: medical/scientific (Prof. Charles Sprung), philosophical/ethical (Prof. Asa Kasher), halakhic (Rabbi Yaakov Ariel), and legal (Prof. Amnon Karmi). The commission consisted of fifty-nine members drawn from various relevant disciplines. All the commissioners were chosen on the strength of their professional qualifications in their respective fields, with no consideration whatever being given to political affiliation, ulterior interests, or public relations.

The subcommittees held a total of thirty-five meetings. After formulation of the draft for the proposed bill, the commission met in three plenary sessions. In all, six different drafts of the bill were discussed.

On January 18, 2002, the proposed law and the commission's report were presented to the minister of health, M.K. Rabbi Nissim Dahan.

CHAPTER 2: THE GUIDING PRINCIPLES

The basic assumption underlying the commission's labors was, for sociological and national reasons, that it was to arrive at ideological and practical solutions regarding the terminally ill patient that would enjoy the widest possible consensus, and that its members would do this by striking a balance between the opposing ideologies at work in the process of decision-making on this subject. There is a unique need for a consensus in the State of Israel, based on its ideological character as a Jewish and democratic state.

The commission set itself the following goals:

1. A proposal comprising a just and fitting balance of all the elements – medical, ethical, religious, socio-psychological, and legal – required for the treatment of the terminally ill patient.

2. A detailed, applicable, and effective draft law, enjoying the widest possible consensus.

The commission examined the legal responses to the plight of the terminally ill patient around the world and found them unsuited to the values of the Jewish and democratic State of Israel. The draft law proposed by the commission is thus largely unique to the State of Israel.

In order to achieve the goals it had set for itself, the commission made a great effort to draft a bill founded on the values of the Jewish and democratic State of Israel, but giving due consideration to the views expressed by representatives of the other faiths in Israel (Christian, Muslim, and Druse).

The draft law is therefore a balance between different values, principally the values of the sanctity of life, prevention of suffering, and respect for the autonomy of the individual. The commission's proposed law is specific to the needs and special values of the State of Israel and consequently contains many unique components and arrangements. The commissioners think that the draft law fulfills most of the requirements – medical, ethical, halakhic, and legal – appertaining to the terminally ill patient, and that it includes suitable mechanisms for the solution of problems not foreseen at present. It is obvious that the draft law, with its many sections, cannot satisfy everybody. Doubtless, too, any draft bill in an area so sensitive and complex will be "rewarded" with criticisms of all sorts (both relevant and otherwise), and no doubt there will be disputes about various sections of the draft law from a variety of standpoints. However, the members of the public commission are of the opinion that the draft law proposed here does represent a just and fitting balance between the various relevant values and between the Israeli public's various approaches, as represented by the members of the commission.

The matter of the terminally ill patient involves several ethical principles:

> The value of life; quality of life; the principle of the patient's autonomy and of his rights; the obligation to benefit one's fellow man and to protect him from harm; just allocation of limited resources.

In addition to these basic principles some further issues must be considered:

> Decisions made under conditions of uncertainty and in face of the possibility of erroneous diagnosis, treatment and prognosis; the duties of the doctor toward the terminally ill patient; the question of the "slippery slope"; the question of the final arbiter; the level of the patient's participation in the decision-making process, the extent of disclosure of information to the patient, and involvement of the family.

More specifically, the public commission's draft law maintains an appropriate balance between the following values:

- The value principle of *the sanctity of life*: this is an attitude to human life based on a normative conception which dictates giving supreme priority to the protection of human life from the threat of all significant danger, immediate or future.
- The importance of *the quality of life*: this is the totality of those aspects of a person's life which have objective value for his health and existence, or subjective value as he or she feels. They depend directly and objectively on the person's physical and mental health, or subjectively on his own estimation of his physical and mental health. The decision should, as far as possible, be made only by the patient, based on his own individual assessment, and not by anyone else.
- The moral value of *preventing significant pain*, pain being the negative experience and sensation, temporary or chronic, with physical characteristics and causes, that stimulate in a person the desire to act and end it speedily and to avoid it as far as possible. Associated with this is the *prevention of suffering*, that is, pain or distress, bodily or mental, which the patient would prefer not to experience by being unconscious, rather than to experience it while conscious; or such pain and distress as a person will make a significant effort to avoid or eliminate.
- The value principle of the dignity of a person and his right to exert his *autonomy*: this is the realization of his power to decide from his own choice whether to act or not, and to decide on matters of principle, be they practical, general, or fundamental, on the basis of his own perception and considerations, as an expression of free will.

All these are discussed in the context of medical care for the terminally ill patient according to the value systems of medicine, ethics, the law, Halakhah and religion.

The draft law deals *comprehensively* with the terminally ill patient and is *limited* to such a patient as defined in the draft law.

The proposed draft law comprises the following elements:

- Definitions relevant to the purposes of this law.
- Fundamental principles.
- Dealing with competent and noncompetent terminally ill patients.
- Dealing with the terminally ill patients of all ages – newborn, minor. and adult.
- Preparation of advance medical directives and appointment of a surrogate
- Status of professional care-givers, family members and friends, religious functionaries, and ethics committees.
- Permitted and prohibited actions in various treatments, including death by omission, known also as merciful death and in the past as passively assisted death (passive euthanasia); this denotes an action purposely omitted, in reasonable expectation that the death of the terminally ill patient will result. Also included is actively assisted death (active euthanasia), where a human action, carried out directly and intentionally, causes accelerated onset of death as a reasonably expected result, even when the action is performed at the wish and the request of the patient.
- Procedures and processes in decision-making.
- Mechanisms for resolving problems by means of institutional and national ethics committees.
- Documentation and control.

The draft law contains some twenty relevant definitions and 115 sections and subsections.

Draft Law: the Terminally Ill Patient, 5762 – 2002

CHAPTER 1: GENERAL PROVISIONS

1. Goal

The purpose of this law is to establish a comprehensive attitude toward the terminally ill patient by establishing a proper balance between the value principle of the sanctity and quality of human life, and between the value principle of a person's dignity and the right to exert his autonomy. This law is based on a system of values – medical, ethical, legal, halakhic, and religious – and on the values of the State of Israel as a democratic Jewish state.

2. Definitions

In this law:

"Care-giver" is a doctor, qualified nurse, social worker, or clinical psychologist.

"Competent person" is a person whose conscious intellectual and mental state allows him to make decisions about medical treatment based on understanding, reasoning, and his own free judgment, and a person who has not been declared legally incompetent.

"Continuous medical treatment" is a medical treatment which, being by nature continuous and uninterrupted, allows of no clear distinction between the end of one cycle of treatment and the beginning of the next and is not planned *a priori* to be given in renewed bouts of treatment.

"Deliberate consent to medical treatment" is defined in the Law on Patients' Rights of 5756/1996.

"Deliberate consent to advance medical directives" is the agreement of a person, given of his own free will, on the basis of medical information as defined in Section 13 of the Law on Patients' Rights, 5756/1996, and of further medical information required by him, and on the basis of his comprehension, deliberation, and decision, on the matter of his wishes to receive or not to receive medical treatment for the medical condition from which he is suffering or will suffer, (the agreement being given) for the event of his not being able formulate or express his will when his condition demands medical treatment for partial or full protection of his life, his health, or the quality of his life.

"Discrete medical treatment" is a medical treatment which, being by nature periodic and interrupted, permits a clear distinction between the end of one cycle of treatment and the beginning of the next and is planned *a priori* to be resumed in renewed bouts of treatment.

"Doctor in charge" is the head of the department or unit responsible for the medical treatment of the terminally ill patient, and likewise a specialist appointed by him for this purpose.

"Incurable medical problem" is an illness, injury, or other bodily dysfunction which is fatal and cannot be cured, arrested, or significantly alleviated in the present state of medical knowledge.

"Life expectancy" is the average duration of life under the given medical circumstances according to modern medical information.

"Medical treatment" is treatment given a person in order to solve a medical problem and based on professional considerations anchored in current medical knowledge according to the principles of medical ethics; a treatment is intended to prolong life, and to improve, correct, alleviate, or cure a pathological or symptomatic condition.

"The minister" is the minister of health, who is appointed to administer this law.

"palliative treatment" is comprehensive treatment given with the main purpose of alleviating a patient's bodily, mental, and existential suffering and of improving the quality of his remaining life.

"Patient at the terminal stage" is a terminally ill patient very close to the final stage, with life expectancy of not more than two weeks, failure of more than one vital bodily system, and significant suffering.

"Personal physician" is a doctor closely acquainted with the patient, his wishes and opinions concerning the medical treatment being given, regardless of whether a family doctor, a doctor appointed by the community, or one personally put in charge of the patient's treatment by the hospital, if so appointed.

"Relative or friend" is a person close to the terminally ill patient by kinship or sentiment, devoted to him and knowing him well through long and continuous contact before or during the medical treatment.

"Significant suffering" is pain or suffering which a reasonable person would try to avoid or to remove with appreciable effort and at considerable cost in quality of life; with regard to an incompetent patient, suffering toward which it is reasonable to suppose that he would so react.

"Special methods of treatment" are methods of medical treatment not routinely used because they are experimental in nature, have a very low chance of success, significantly increase suffering, or are likely to cause significant harm to the recipient of the treatment or to others.

"Surrogate" is someone explicitly appointed by a person under Section 16 of the Law on Patients' Rights of 5756/1996, after due consideration and deliberation, in order to decide in that person's stead on future medical treatment or omission of treatment, in the event of his becoming incompetent to give instructions.

"Terminally ill patient" is a patient suffering from an incurable medical condition, whose life expectancy is no more than half a year in the present state of medical knowledge.

3. Applicability

(a) The provisions of this law shall apply only to the terminally ill patient.

(b) The doctor in charge is authorized to determine, in consultation with the specialists of the treating team, whether the medical condition of the patient satisfies the definition of a terminally ill patient. If the personal physician of the patient is available, he is also to be consulted.

(c) If the patient or his surrogate disagrees with the determination made by the doctor in charge, the institution's ethics committee shall adjudicate.

4. Obligatory consultation

Once the patient has been determined to be terminally ill, the doctor in charge and the treating team shall, as soon as possible, hold a comprehensive conference on the condition of the patient and on the medical treatment appropriate to his case, in accord with the provisions of this law.

CHAPTER 2: PRINCIPLES AND PRESUMPTIONS

5. Basic Principle

The medical condition, wishes, and significant suffering of the terminally ill patient are exclusively the data for deciding on the further treatment or nontreatment of the patient..

6. The Presumption of the Will to Live

(a) It is presumed that a person wishes to continue living unless there is proof beyond all doubt to the contrary; in the event of doubt, the option of life is to be favored.

(b) The presumption of the patient's will to live is abandoned only if one of the following holds true:

  (1) for a competent patient – according to his latest utterance.

  (2) for a noncompetent patient –

    (a) according to advance medical directives or according to

the directives of his surrogate, in accord with the provisions in Chapter 4 of this law.

(b) In the absence of advance medical directives or of a surrogate, the doctor in charge must make every effort to obtain the testimony of a relative or friend as defined above, and the doctor in charge is allowed to take into account their clear testimony.

(3) In the absence of all these, the doctor may take into consideration the opinion of a guardian, if such has been appointed.

(c) The duty of a care-giver to do everything in his power to save the life of a patient and to delay his death is not binding in the case of a terminally ill patient for whom the presumption of the will to live has been abandoned, when the treatment is likely to prolong suffering; and all as stated in this law.

7. The Presumption of Competence

(a) A person is presumed to be competent; this presumption applies to a person who has reached the age of seventeen.

(b) No person is to be denied the presumption of competence for the purposes of this law except by the authoritative, reasoned, and documented medical decision of the doctor in charge, in consultation with the care-giving team.

(c) If the decision of the doctor in charge is unacceptable to the patient, the institution's ethics committee shall adjudicate.

(d) As to a minor of under seventeen years, the care-giving team shall assess his competence and intellectual and mental maturity, and in accord with their findings engage him in the decision about further treatment. If there is disagreement between the minor and his parents or between the former and the care-giving team, the institution's ethics committee shall adjudicate.

8. The Presumption of Validity

An advance medical directive remains in force until it is proven that the attitude of its author has changed.

CHAPTER 3: TREATMENT OF THE
TERMINALLY ILL PATIENT

ARTICLE 1: THE TERMINALLY ILL PATIENT WHO WISHES TO
CONTINUE LIVING

9. (a) If a competent terminally ill patient requests medical treatment
beyond what is proposed by the care-giving team for prolonging his
life, the team is obliged to accede to this request, except for treatment
which, on medical assessment, is not expected to prolong the patient's
life or treatment which might cause significant harm to the patient.

 (b) As to a noncompetent patient –

> (1) his advance medical directives, or the directive of his sur-
> rogate in accordance with Chapter 4 of this law, or the direc-
> tive of his guardian, or the joint, unambiguous, and lucid
> testimony of relatives and friends shall be regarded as express-
> ing the wishes of the terminally ill patient in this matter. The
> doctor in charge may regard the clearly expressed testimony
> of a single relative or friend of the terminally ill patient as ex-
> pressing the latter's will in this matter.
> (2) The doctor in charge must make a reasonable effort to
> obtain all the data and documents from the relevant parties
> as in Subsection (1) above and to reach agreement on the
> further treatment of the terminally ill patient. In the event of
> disagreement between the above parties or between the doc-
> tor in charge and the said parties, the decision shall lie with
> the institution's ethics committee or with the latter's autho-
> rized delegate in accordance with Article 1 of Chapter 5 of this
> Law.

ARTICLE 2: THE TERMINALLY ILL PATIENT WHO DOES NOT
DESIRE PROLONGATION OF HIS LIFE

10. Medical treatment for the competent terminally ill patient
A terminally ill patient who is no longer presumed to be desirous of
living according to Section 6(b) above and is competent –

(a) shall not be given medical treatment unless he has given his deliberate consent;

(b) it is the medical team's duty to make all efforts to persuade the patient to accept oxygen, food, drink, regular medication, and palliative treatment in some form unless there are medical counter-indications.

11. Medical treatment for the noncompetent terminally ill patient

A terminally ill patient who is no longer presumed to be desirous of living under Section 6(b) above and is not competent, shall be given medical treatment –

(a) according to advance medical directives or the directives of a surrogate as in the rulings of Chapter 4.

(b) In the absence of advance medical directive or the directives of a surrogate, the medical team may consider the testimony of a relative or friend of the terminally ill patient with regard to the latter's wishes concerning medical treatment to be given, or the opinion of a guardian, should there be one. The doctor in charge must make a reasonable effort to obtain all the data and documents from all these relevant parties and to come to an agreement about the further medical treatment of the terminally ill patient.

(c) In the event of disagreement between the above parties or between the doctor in charge and any of the said parties, the decision shall lie with the institution's ethics committee or with the latter's authorized delegate in accordance with Section 1 of Chapter 5 of this law.

(d) In the absence of these data or documents, and when the case is one of a noncompetent terminally ill patient in the terminal stage, the doctor may act in accordance with the rulings of this law in Sections 12 to 13 and may also refrain from special methods of treatment.

12. Interruption of Medical Treatment

(a) It is forbidden to interrupt a continuous medical treatment for purposes other than medical treatment if the interruption is likely to bring about the death of the patient, be he competent or noncompetent. However, it is permitted to interrupt a discrete medical treatment, subject to Section 13.

(b) A continuous medical treatment interrupted purely for medical reasons shall be subject to Section 13(a).

13. Refraining from Medical Treatment

(a) Subject to the provisions of this law, medical treatment related to the terminally ill patient's incurable medical problem, whether he be competent or not, need not be undertaken if the treatment involves considerable suffering. Likewise, one may refrain from resuscitation, connection to a respirator, chemotherapy or radiotherapy, dialysis, surgery, examinations, and experimental treatments.

(b) As to a noncompetent terminally ill patient, it is forbidden to refrain from treatments directed at medical events other than his incurable condition, that is, routine treatments necessitated by intercurrent disorders, background disorders, and pain. It is forbidden to withhold food and drink in any manner.

(c) The prohibition of Subsection 13(b) above shall not apply if there are proven medical contraindications for the patient; nor shall they apply if there exist advance medical directives which require that such treatments be withheld. However, advance medical directives to desist from such treatments shall not be valid except for a patient at a terminal stage, when the issue is one of food, drink, or routine treatments, the withholding of which is not expected to cause an immediate curtailment of the life of the terminally ill patient.

14. Medical Emergency

(a) In a medical emergency affecting a noncompetent terminally ill patient, or when his attitude cannot be ascertained because of the emergency and he has not given advance expression to his wishes in one of the forms required by this law, and in the absence of clear testimony from a relative or friend, the procedure shall be as dictated by Section 15(3) of the Law of Patient's Rights of 5756/1996.

(b) As to a patient, recognized by the doctor to be at the terminal stage, who is in a state of medical emergency under the conditions described in Subsection (a) above, the doctor is permitted to refrain from life-saving medical treatment and is also permitted to refrain from special methods of treatment.

15. Palliative Treatment
(a) The purpose of palliative treatment is to alleviate pain and suffering, and to improve the quality of life.
(b) It is the duty of the care-giving team to do all they can to alleviate the pain and suffering of the terminally ill patient, whether he be competent or not, despite some reasonable risk to his life, by means of pain-killing or other appropriate drugs, or by psychological, nursing, or environmental means, in accordance with the principles and norms accepted in palliative treatment.
(c) The care-giving team must also work as far as possible for the welfare of the members of the terminally ill patient's family, in accordance with the principles and norms accepted in social and palliative care.

16. Prohibition of Actively Assisted Death
An act which is medical treatment, or appears to be a medical treatment, whose purpose or whose certain outcome, according to the majority of contemporary expert opinion in the field, is homicidal, is also forbidden if the act will be carried out from motives of kindness and compassion, or is carried out at the explicit request of the terminally ill patient, his surrogate, guardian, relative, friend, or any other person.

17. Assisted Suicide
Assistance to suicide by a care-giver or any other person is forbidden also when carried out from motives of kindness and compassion and also if at the explicit request of the terminally ill patient.

ARTICLE 3: DOCUMENTATION AND ASSESSMENT

18. The Obligation to Record
As soon as the method by which the terminally ill patient is to be medically treated has been decided –

(a) the doctor in charge must record the discussion, arguments, and decisions in the file of the terminally ill patient;

(b) the doctor in charge must make a reasonable effort to inform, immediately and clearly, those relevant parties known to him, doctors and others involved in the care of the terminally ill patient, and must also permit the involved parties to inspect the medical information, unless the terminally ill patient has forbidden any of them to receive medical information about himself. Contravening rules of medical secrecy shall not apply with regard to this paragraph.

(c) The minister shall establish procedural rules of standard recording and reporting procedures for making decisions as they affect the terminally ill patient under this law, for control and research purposes both at the level of the patient's medical records and at the national level, and for informing the parties involved in the treatment of the patient about the decision.

19. The Obligation of Repeat Assessment

Assessment of the terminally ill patient must be carried out repeatedly, and when a change occurs in his condition or his wishes, the strategy of medical treatment for the patient must be redetermined.

CHAPTER 4: ASCERTAINING THE WISHES OF THE NONCOMPETENT PATIENT

20. General Remarks

(a) A person may in advance express his will as regards the medical treatment which he shall or shall not be given in the event of terminal illness, and this by issuing advance medical directives or by appointing a surrogate, or by a combination of these, according to the provisions of this chapter.

(b) Documented advance medical directives and the directives of a surrogate are binding, subject to the provisions of this law.

ARTICLE 1: ADVANCE MEDICAL DIRECTIVES

21. Fundamental Provisions

Advance medical directives are an instrument for the manifestation of a person's desire to exert his autonomy, within the permitted limits of this law, when he is no longer fit or able to express this desire. The validity of the directives shall accord with the provisions of this law.

22. Competence to Issue Directives

A person at least seventeen years of age who is competent to give considered consent to medical directives is competent to issue them.

23. Insignificance of Directives Not Given

The fact that a person has not issued advance medical directives shall have no significance as to his wishes concerning medical care.

24. The Preparation and Documentation of Directives

Advance medical directives may be recorded in a formula to be fixed by regulation or in some other formula, or by other technical means. Advance medical directives which have not been documented are not binding, but they are to be taken into account among the deliberations of those making the decisions, in accordance with Section 9.

25. Conditions for the Validity of the Directives

(a) Advance medical directives shall be valid if they are issued by their author after receiving the necessary medical information from a doctor or a qualified nurse. The directives shall be signed by their author and by two witnesses, and the doctor or qualified nurse may serve as a witness.

(b) The advance medical directives document shall include the essential medical information given to the person prior to his signing the document and a declaration that his advance medical directives were given freely, based on comprehension, deliberation, and decision.

26. Commencement of the Directives' Validity

The advance medical directives shall come into force at a time when the terminally ill patient has lost the competence or the ability to express his wishes concerning the medical treatment, and they shall remain in force as long as the terminally ill patient remains deprived of the said competence or ability.

27. Directives Which Are Unclear or Inappropriate

If the wishes of the terminally ill patient do not emerge clearly from the advance medical directives which he issued, or if these directives do not suit the circumstances, or if they severely offend human dignity, then – in the absence of a surrogate, a guardian, or the clear testimony of a relative or friend – the institution's ethics committee shall adjudicate.

28. Directives Concerning Preservation of the Patient's Autonomy

Special advance medical directives enshrining their author's concepts of personal dignity, which he is allowed to issue as a competent person, shall be binding.

ARTICLE 2: THE SURROGATE

29. Empowerment

(a) A person may appoint any other person competent to act as surrogate to make decisions in his stead concerning his medical treatment for the purposes of this law. The empowerment shall be subject to the provisions of Section 16 of the Law on Patients' Rights of 5756/1996 and on the provisions of this Article.

(b) A person may appoint a substitute surrogate who shall fulfill this task if the surrogate is unable to, or prevented from doing so.

30. Methods of Appointment

(a) The empowerment of surrogates shall be documented, with the signature of the appointer and two witnesses.

(b) The appointer must state explicitly in the letter of appointment that the surrogate shall be authorized to take decisions in his stead in the matter of his medical treatment if he, as a terminally ill patient, becomes incompetent or unable to express his will by himself.

(c) The appointer shall enumerate in detail in the document of appointment, the circumstances and conditions under which the surrogate shall be authorized to decide in the appointer's stead about the medical treatments, all or in part.

31. Validity of the Appointment

The validity of the surrogates' authority is from the time they received the appointment or from a time specified by the appointer in the letter of appointment.

32. Authority

The authority of surrogates is limited to actions which are permitted by this law.

33. Appeal against the Surrogate's Decision

A person who suspects that the surrogate is not acting according to the wishes of the terminally ill patient or not to his benefit, or is acting out of a conflict of interests, may apply to the institutional ethics committee in order to obtain its decision as to medical treatment appropriate for the terminally ill patient.

ARTICLE 3: COMBINATION OF ADVANCE MEDICAL DIRECTIVES AND THE APPOINTMENT OF A SURROGATE

34. Possibility of Combination

A person may combine advance medical directives given under Article 1 with the appointment of a surrogate to act on his behalf under Article 2 above.

35. Priorities

(a) The advance medical directives and the letter of appointment of the surrogate may include instructions concerning the priorities of the directives in the event of a clash between an advance medical directive and a directive of the surrogate.

(b) In the absence of defined priorities between the advance medical directives and the directives of the surrogate, if these were given in association, or if the advance medical directive was made later than the appointment, the advance medical directive takes precedence; if the appointment was made after the advance medical directive, the institutional ethics committee shall adjudicate.

ARTICLE 4: GENERAL DIRECTIVES

36: Annulment and Changes

(a) Advance medical directives or the appointment of a surrogate can be changed or annulled by their author at any time and in any of the manners by which they are initially made.

(b) Decisions as to annulment of or changes in advance medical directives or the appointment of surrogates shall be recorded in writing in advance, or if subsequently, then immediately or at the earliest opportunity.

37. Precedence of the Explicit Will

The explicit wishes of the terminally ill patient, when he is competent, take precedence over any advance medical directives he issued in the past, any directive given by his surrogates or guardian, and any testimony given by a relation or friend concerning any medical treatment.

38. The Database and Renewal of Directives

(a) The minister shall be responsible for the establishment of a central database in which all advance medical directives and appointments of surrogates will be recorded.

(b) The minister will determine directives concerning methods of documentation in the central database. He will also determine directives about access to the data in the central database. The provisions of the Law on Defense of Privacy shall apply to the central database.

(c) Every five years, the managers of the database shall send out reminders to renew or bring up to date the advance medical directives or appointments of surrogates, in order to maintain their validity.

(d) If the advance medical directives were not renewed even though the author received a reminder, they are presumed to testify to the patient's wishes.

39. Documentation in the Medical File

A person is entitled to request that his advance medical directives or the appointment he made be recorded in his medical file as kept by the Health Fund of which he is a member, or in the hospital in which he is being treated, and the medical institution must act according to his request.

40. Efforts to Ascertain the Existence of Advance Medical Directives or of a Surrogate

(a) When a person who is evidently a terminally ill patient arrives at a hospital for medical treatment or as an in-patient, the treating team is obliged to make a reasonable effort to find out if the terminally ill patient has issued advance medical directives or has appointed a surrogate, and if this is the case, the doctor shall attach this information to the medical file being kept on the patient.

(b) At the first opportunity arising for the doctor to act according to the advance medical directives, the patient, if he is competent, shall be asked by the doctor in charge to confirm or bring up to date the advance medical directives, and this after the medical information has been given him by a doctor or by a qualified nurse in the presence of a doctor.

41. The Obligation to Inform

(a) The treating doctor shall inform the surrogate, guardian, relation, or friend of his intention to act according to the advance medical directives the terminally ill patient issued, and shall make them privy to the medical information.

(b) The treating doctor shall inform the relation or friend of his intention to act according to the directives of the surrogate or guardian, unless the patient forbade such information to be passed to them.

(c) In the absence of advance medical directives, a surrogate, or a guardian, the doctor shall make the relative or friend privy to the planned treatment of the terminally ill patient, unless the patient has forbidden such information to be passed to them.

(d) Contravening rules of medical secrecy shall not apply to this Section.

CHAPTER 5: INFANTS AND MINORS

42. Infants

43. Minors

Infants and minors wore not dealt with by the commission. Section 42 and 43 were therefore left empty and to be completed by a later commission.

CHAPTER 6: ETHICS COMMITTEES

44. Committees

Ethics committees shall be set up at the institutional and national levels in accordance with this law, and these will function as ethics committees in the sense of the Law of Patients' Rights, 1996/5756.

ARTICLE 1: INSTITUTIONAL ETHICS COMMITTEE

45. Composition of the Committee and Appointment of its Members

(a) An institutional ethics committee shall be made up of representatives of the following occupations:

- Four doctors, not part of the team treating the terminally ill pa-

tient, representing medical specializations from among the following: internal medicine, geriatrics, cardiology, neurology, oncology, palliative medicine, intensive care, anesthetics, psychiatry, family medicine. In the case of a child, one of the four specialists shall be a pediatrician, and in the case of an infant, one of the four specialists shall be neonatologist;
- a qualified nurse;
- a social worker or a clinical psychologist;
- an ethicist;
- a lawyer
- a rabbi, or in the event of the terminally ill patient being a non-Jew, a religious figure from the same religious community as the terminally ill patient.

(b) An institutional ethics committee shall elect its chairman.

(c) The patient or his agent may request the participation in the deliberations of the institutional committee of a representative who reflects the patient's values. This representative shall have the right to vote.

(d) The patient or his agent are entitled to appear before the committee in order to present their arguments, The patient and this agent shall not have the right to vote.

(e) The members of the institutional ethics committee shall be appointed by the director of the hospital in consultation with the chairman of the National Ethics Committee and with the approval of the director of the Ministry of Health.

(f) The institutional ethics committee may authorize a narrower forum from among its members to discuss specific cases if the need arises for urgent discussion. The narrow forum must contain a physician and another two members, chosen from the following: a lawyer, an ethicist, and a religious figure.

(g) The members of an institutional ethics committee shall take intensive courses in order to familiarize themselves with this law and its background and with the Law on Patients' Rights of 5756/1996. The director of the Ministry of Health is responsible for organizing the courses.

46. APPEALS TO THE COMMITTEE

- Any one of the following parties may appeal to the institutional ethics committee:
  - the terminally ill patient himself if he is competent, or the surrogate of a competent terminally ill patient who is suffering from physical limitations;
  - the surrogate, guardian, relation, or friend of a noncompetent terminally ill patient;
  - a care-giver from the medical team.

47. ADJUDICATION BY THE COMMITTEE

(a) An institutional ethics committee is authorized to adjudicate in cases of doubt as to handling a terminally ill patient or in cases of dispute between the parties involved as to handling a terminally ill patient, and all this subject to the provisions of this law. In particular the institutional ethics committee shall discuss the issues detailed in Sections 3(c), 7(c), 7(d), 33, 35(b), and 55(b).

(b) The goal underlying the decisions of the institutional ethics committee is to clarify and put into effect the wishes of the terminally ill patient concerning his medical treatment, on the basis of the factual data presented to it.

(c) In the absence of factual data, the institutional ethics committee shall reach its decision by assessing the patient's wishes according to his outlook on life and his life-style, if necessary in consultation with people of similar *Weltanschauung* if it is not represented on the committee.

(d) The decisions of the institutional ethics committee shall be taken on the opinion of the majority.

(e) The decisions of the institutional ethics committee shall be valid only if five members have taken part in the debate and voting, among them being at least one who is a physician and two who are not physicians.

(f) The institutional ethics committee may determine that its decision is binding or that it is merely a recommendation upon which the care-giver is to act.

ARTICLE 2: NATIONAL ETHICS COMMITTEE

48. Powers of the Committee

(a) A National Ethics Committee is authorized to adjudicate in cases where there are unresolved differences of opinion in the institutional ethics committee, or in cases of an appeal against the decision of an institutional ethics committee and in exceptional cases involving important principles.

(b) The main goal of the National Ethics Committee is to clarify and put into effect the wishes of the terminally ill patient concerning his medical treatment, on the basis of the factual data with which it will be presented.

(c) In the absence of factual data, the National Ethics Committee shall assess the presumed wishes of the patient according to his outlook on life and his life-style, if necessary in consultation with people of a similar *Weltanschauung* if it is not represented on the committee during its deliberations.

49. Composition of the Committee and Appointment of Its Members

(a) The National Ethics Committee shall be made up of representatives of the following occupations with experience in the areas relevant to this law:

- a doctor ranking as head of unit, head of department, or hospital director;
- an ethicist of senior academic rank;
- a rabbi of senior rabbinical rank. For cases involving non-Jewish patients, a religious figure of senior rank in the relevant religious community;
- a lawyer with the qualifications of a High Court judge or one of senior academic rank;
- a qualified nurse of senior managerial rank;
- a hospital social worker of senior managerial rank or a hospital clinical psychologist of senior managerial rank.

At their first appointment, all these shall be in active professional service or no more than five years after the conclusion of such service.
(b) The appointment shall be for five years, renewable for a further five years.
(c) Four persons shall be appointed in each profession represented on the National Committee; and one representative from each profession and a deputy shall be invited to take part in its deliberations.
(d) There must be appropriate representation of men and women on the committee.
(e) The director of the Ministry of Health shall appoint the chairman of the National Ethics Committee and his deputy.
(f) The members of the National Ethics Committees shall be appointed by the director of the Ministry of Health. The rabbi shall be appointed in consultation with the Chief Rabbis of Israel; the non-Jewish senior religious figure shall be appointed in consultation with the president of the Appeals Court of the appropriate religious denomination in Israel; the lawyer shall be appointed in consultation with the attorney-general.
(g) The patient or his surrogate may appoint a spokesman to the National Ethics Committee who reflects the patient's values. This appointee shall have the right to vote.
(h) The patient or his surrogate may appear before the committee in order to make their pleas. Neither the patient nor his surrogate shall have the right to vote.

50. Adjudication by the Committee
(a) The decisions of the National Ethics Committee shall be taken on the opinion of the majority.
(b) The decisions of the National Ethics Committee shall be binding.
(c) The validity of the National Ethics Committee's decisions is conditional on the participation in the discussions of a representative of every profession making up the committee.

51. Appeals to the Committee

(a) Any one of the following parties may appeal to the National Ethics Committee:

- the terminally ill patient himself if he is competent, or the surrogate of a competent terminally ill patient who is suffering from physical limitations;
- the surrogate, guardian, relation, or friend of a noncompetent terminally ill patient;
- a care-giver from the medical team
- any member of an institutional ethics committee.

(b) In all cases, appeal to the National Ethics Committee shall be permitted only after debate in an institutional ethics committee, unless the case is exceptional in the importance of the principles involved, when a direct appeal to the National Ethics Committee is allowable.

52. Appeal

Any one of the parties with the right to appeal to the National Ethics Committee is entitled to appeal its decision before a District Court panel of three judges.

CHAPTER 7: MISCELLANEOUS

53. Exemption from Legal Liability

A care-giver and a member of an ethics committee shall not be legally liable for their action when these accord with the provisions of this law.

54. The Right to Consultation

(a) A terminally ill patient is entitled to instruct the treating team to transfer medical information to persons whom he wishes to involve in his decisions, within the limits of the law and of medical ethics.

(b) A terminally ill patient is entitled to request the cooperation of the treating team in unconventional treatment, subject to approval by the director of the hospital.

55. Transfer of Treatment to Another Care-Giver for Reasons of Conscience

(a) The provisions of this law do not oblige a care-giver to provide medical treatment to a terminally ill patient or to refrain from doing so, against his values, conscience, or medical judgment, but he must transfer treatment of the patient to another care-giver by a procedure to be prearranged with the management of the hospital.

(b) A care-giver who is opposed in principle to the treatment of the terminally ill patient in accordance with the provisions of this law may be relieved by the institutional ethics committee, at his request, of the duty to treat the terminally ill patient medically when he is opposed on the grounds of values or conscience to carrying out the directives included in this law as regards the treatment or nontreatment of an terminally ill patient, but only if a proper alternative is found for the medical treatment of the terminally ill patient within the provisions of the law. The committee may refuse this only if no proper alternative medical treatment can be proposed for the patient within the provisions of this law.

EXCERPTS FROM THE DISCUSSIONS ON THE DRAFT LAW: CONTROVERSY AND CONSENSUS AMONG THE MEMBERS OF THE COMMISSION

Sections 12 and 13 (on refraining from and terminating treatments) are of particular interest because they aroused the greatest divergence of opinion. The discussion on these two sections is reported in full.

For convenience, the two sections are cited again, with the ensuing comments:

12. Interruption of Medical Treatment

(a) It is forbidden to interrupt a continuous medical treatment for purposes other than medical treatment if the interruption is likely to bring about the death of the patient, be he competent or noncompetent. However, it is permitted to interrupt a discrete medical treatment, subject to Section 13.

(b) A continuous medical treatment that was interrupted purely for medical reasons shall be subject to Section 13(a).

Note:

(a) The main relevant treatment, indeed almost the only one to be included in the definition of continuous medical treatment, is artificial respiration (with a ventilator or respirator). In contrast, almost all relevant treatments of the terminally ill patient are included in the definition of a discrete medical treatment, examples being chemotherapy, radiotherapy, dialysis, and ther like. See also the note after Article 13.

(b) The interruption of a respirator for medical reasons refers to circumstances where there are medical data allowing the patient to be weaned off the respirator as part of a medical procedure on the assumption that the patient will continue to live without resort to respiration. If, in the course of weaning and the period immediately thereafter, the patient remains stable according to the vital signs, and his condition subsequently becomes more severe or deteriorates, Article 13(a) shall apply.

13. REFRAINING FROM MEDICAL TREATMENT

(a) Subject to the contents of this law, medical treatment related to the terminally ill patient's incurable medical problem, whether he be competent or not, need not be undertaken if the treatment involves considerable suffering. Likewise, one may refrain from resuscitation, connection to a respirator, chemotherapy or radiotherapy, dialysis, surgery, examinations, and experimental treatments.

(b) As to a noncompetent terminally ill patient, it is forbidden to refrain from treatments directed at medical events other than his incurable condition, that is, routine treatments necessitated by intercurrent disorders, background disorders, and pain. It is forbidden in any manner to withhold food and drink.

(c) The prohibition in Subsection 13(b) above shall not apply if there are proven medical contraindications for the patient; nor shall they apply if there exist advance medical directives which require that such treatments be withheld. However, advance medical directives to desist from such treatments shall not be valid except for a patient at a terminal stage, when the issue is one of food, drink, or routine treatments, the withholding of which is not expected to cause a curtailment of the life of the terminally ill patient.

Note:
(a) Sections 12 and 13 refer to a circumstance which used to be called "euthanasia," "passive death," or "passively assisted death" ("passive euthanasia"). These terms are controversial in the professional literature, so the majority of members of the public commission decided not to include them in Section 2, Definitions, but instead to refer to the realities as described in Sections 12 and 13.
(b) These sections aroused the most controversy among the commission's members, and some rejected them. The above proposal is based on a series of presumptions, as follows:

> The proponents of the value of life as an absolute and infinite value cannot agree to the limitation of any treatment, whether it is continuous or discrete, whether it is to be interrupted or withheld, whether the treatment is directed at the incurable condition or whether it is routine. In their opinion, treatment to prolong the life of the patient must be continued irrespective of the quality of life or its expected length, and irrespective also of the patient's wishes or his refusal in the matter. The proponents of autonomy as a supreme or even absolute value cannot agree to any limitation on the wishes of the patients in anything that concerns his treatment. Thus they too do not distinguish at all between forms of treatment, except that in this view, every treatment should be dispensed with or stopped, whether it relates to the incurable disease or not, and even food and drink – all being subject to the wishes of the patient. Moreover, in the extreme form of the principle of autonomy, the patient's wish for assisted suicide or even for actively assisted death should be respected. All the members of the commission agreed that the balance had to be found between the value of life and that of autonomy. Therefore they all agreed

that the autonomic request by a terminally ill patient to be put to death is not be granted (Section 16 above), and almost all agreed that the wish of a terminally ill patient for assistance with suicide is not to be granted (Section 17 above). On the other hand, all the members of the commission agreed that not every patient should be treated without limit and against his will. But disagreement remained among the members of the public commission about the details of the balance between these extremes: Some commissioners thought that the correct balance lies in respecting the value of life in all that concerns actively assisted death and assisted suicide while respecting the value of autonomy in all that concerns all treatments and modes of treatment. Thus, in their opinion, actively assisted death or assisted suicide is to be forbidden even when either is the wish of the patient. Yet his wish for no treatment is to be respected, without distinction between continuous or discrete treatment, or between treatment of his incurable condition or otherwise, since, in their opinion, these distinctions have no moral basis, and no treatment or its continuation should be imposed on any person against their will. Opposing them were commission members who opined that there is a legal and moral difference between refraining passively from an action, as in the talmudic phrase "sit and do nothing," even if this results in the death of the patient, albeit from his sickness and not by human intervention, and between the positive action of disconnecting an apparatus, as in the contrasting phrase "go and act," where the action itself brings about the patient's death. Some commissioners thought that there is also a difference, from an emotional and professional standpoint, between refraining from treatment and interrupting it, as has indeed emerged from opinion polls among doctors and nurses, who make the distinction between these two modes in practice. Other members of the commission thought that, although morally speaking there was no difference between withholding and interrupting a treatment, medical ethics nevertheless demands that a distinction be made between them, since it is the physician's task to heal and to save lives and not to shorten them. Thus, the actual and manual interruption of treatment is a breach of medical ethics. Some other commissioners feared the "slippery slope" whereby the permission to interrupt continuous treatment will bring in its train the permission for actively assisted death and assisted suicide, because of the great practical similarity between these categories.

Some of the commission members made a distinction between treatments of incurable conditions, for which one could impose limitations according to the stipulations of this law, and treatments unconnected with the incurable disorder, because forgoing treatment for these unconnected disorders, and certainly forgoing food and drink, is, in fact, a form of suicide. As some members put it: "This was hitching a ride on the treatment of the incurable disease in order to get to death." Some members did not see the terminal-stage medical treatments as a package-deal, as "all or nothing," but distinguished between different treatments. Others distinguished between medical treatments and the supply of food and drink. The latter are, in their opinion, basic human needs and should not be regarded as forms of treatment Withholding them, and consequent death from hunger and thirst constitute a significant offense to human dignity.

(c) It emerged at all events that the approach which does not distinguish between types of treatment and between the ways they are administered or not administered is diametrically opposed to the halakhic position as expressed by the overwhelming majority of deciding authorities (*poskim*). According to this position, the interruption of a continuous procedure that leads to the death of the patient is tantamount to homicide and is legally to be considered as actively assisted death (Section 16 above). Similarly, forgoing food and drink and routine treatment is within the definition of suicide and is therefore forbidden (Section 17 above). On the other hand, many *poskim*, though not all, agree that it is permissible to refrain from treatment of an incurable condition. One opinion holds that this is permissible only if the treatment itself causes exacerbated and fresh suffering for the patient. But many *poskim* hold that the actual prolongation of a suffering life is cause for desisting from medical efforts aimed at the incurable sickness.

(d) The presumption of the commission's members was that the bone of contention, the interruption of a respirator, is of likely practical relevance to a limited number of cases. A person who desires this procedure, also during subsequent treatment as a terminally ill patient, is certainly entitled to it. A person who does not desire this treatment as a terminally ill patient can forgo the treatment in accord with this law in a number of ways; a terminally ill patient at the terminal stage shall not be connected to the respirator unless he requests it. Thus, the number of cases for which any need will arise for disconnection of a terminally ill patient from a respirator is expected to be small. At the same time, the members of the commission agreed that a proper solution must be found also for these patients, and their cases can be heard by the National Ethics Committee on the strength of its authority to consider exceptional cases that involve significant matters of principle (Section 48(a) above). Under various conditions, a continuous procedure can also be turned into a discrete one, as by the installation of a timer on the respirator, or by other means which will be examined in the near future by experts in medical technology and put into practice as soon as possible. See also Chapter 5 of the commission's report, for recommendations by the public commission's members in this matter. One commissioner pointed out that one *posek* does not accept the timer solution because of possible mishaps, although most *poskim* opine that this solution is halakhahally acceptable.

RECOMMENDATIONS ARISING OUT OF
THE DEBATES ON THE DRAFT LAW

- Establishment of a special control procedure to check on the care of terminally ill patients, underlying considerations, discussions by the care-giving team, discussions by the institutional ethics committees, and documentation.
- Encouragement of palliative treatment, including recognition of this field as a medical specialization; teaching palliative medicine in medical schools to students and interns, and in postgraduate

courses; training of specialists in palliative medicine; establishment of hospices and of home care; enhanced awareness by doctors of the general principles of palliative medical treatment.
- Instruction in the ethics of care for terminally ill patients to be given in appropriate teaching environments,such as medical school, postgraduate medical courses, nursing school, legal and philosophical studies, and so on.
- Changes in the composition of the ethics committee and its functions as defined in the Law on Patients' Rights in order to conform with those proposed in this law, with consequent unification of these committees.
- Innovation of a document for advance medical directives and a document for the proper appointment of a surrogate, and the recommendation that these documents should be freely available to the public in hospitals and clinics.
- The training of doctors and nurses in the qualification to guide people in issuing advance medical directives.
- Establishment of a technical commission to develop a device (such as a timer) suitable for converting continuous treatment with an artificial respirator into a discrete treatment.

In December 2005 the proposed law was finally approved by the Knesset without significant changes.

Glossary

Aggadah The narrative and allegorical passages in the Talmud.

Ashkenazic Jews Jews originating from central and eastern Europe (Ashkenaz is Hebrew for Germany)

Assisted death Sometimes called euthanasia. Deeds of commission or omission that take into account, or have as their aim, the possible or certain curtailment of a terminal patient's life or the induction of his demise.

Baraita Oral Law material that existed at the time of the Mishnah but was not included therein.

B.C.E. Before the common era.

Brain death Complete failure of all brain functions under circumstances when pulse and breathing can still be maintained for a certain time by artificial means. It is accepted in modern medicine as "clinical death" but is not accepted as death by some groups, including some ultra-Orthodox Jews.

BT Babylonian Talmud.

C.E. Common era

End-of-life patient Patient suffering from an incurable and fatal disorder who is in the last months of life.

Final-stage patient Terminal patient in the last days of life.

Goses A dying person; according to talmudic definition, somebody whose life expectancy is less than three days.

Halakhah Lit. "the (right) way"; Jewish religious law. Because the Talmud and Midrash often differ or contradict one other on certain points, an authoritative codification of Jewish law has been sought for over a thousand years. The last attempt, accepted as binding to this day, was made by Joseph Caro in the sixteenth century and is called the *Bet Yosef*, better known in its abbreviated form, the *Shulhan Arukh*.

Hilkhot Commentary, explanation.

JT Jerusalem Talmud.

Masorah Tradition.

Midrash (pl. Midrashim) Commentaries from talmudic and post-talmudic times.

Mishnah A postbiblical, very briefly formulated collection of laws. Transmitted orally for centuries, it was edited and committed to writing in the second century C.E.

Olam ha-ba The hereafter, lit. "the World to Come."

Pikuah nefesh A life-threatening danger.

Posek (pl. poskim) A respected rabbi who makes halakhic decisions (*see also* Responsum).

Persistent and permanent vegetative state (PVS) A vegetative state is a coma following hypoxic brain damage caused by disease or injury. There is no tangible perception. A vegetative state that lasts over a month is called persistent. If it is most probably irreversible, it is called a permanent vegetative status.

Rambam The Hebrew acronym for Rabbi Moses ben Maimon, also known as Maimonides, probably the most famous Jewish talmudic scholar, philosopher, and physician of the Middle Ages (1135–1205). Author of an important halakhic code, the *Mishneh Torah*, also known as the *Yad Hazakah*.

Rabbi, Rav A Jewish teacher or religious leader; the word derives from *rav* = much, i.e., one who knows much.

Regesh Feeling, empathy

Responsum Rabbinic reply to a halakhic query (*see also* Posek).

Sephardic Jews Jews originating from the western part of the medieval Islamic empire whose center was in Spain (Hebrew: Sefarad). After the Jews were expelled from Spain in 1492, they resettled mainly around the Mediterranean basin in

Turkey, the Balkans, and North Africa. Jews originating from the eastern medieval Islamic empire (Middle East, Persia) are also (incorrectly) included in this term.

Shulhan Arukh Authoritative codification of the Halakhah by Rabbi Joseph Caro (1488–1575), Safed, now always published with annotations by Rabbi Moses Isserles (1525–1572), Cracow, Poland.

Suicide aid, Assisted suicide Preparation or prescription of a lethal substance in order to enable a person to commit suicide.

Talmud Vast body of rabbinic commentary and discussion (Gemara) on the Mishnah; also known as the Oral Law because it was transmitted orally for centuries. Its composition was finalized in the sixth century (Babylonian Talmud) and fourth century (Jerusalem Talmud).

Tanna, pl. tannaim Earliest generation of Talmud scholars, from the first century B.C.E. to the second century C.E.

Terminal sedation Deliberate and final elimination or severe dimming of the consciousness of a dying person, induced by sedatives.

Theonomy Knowledge about God; the study of God's being.

Terminally sick, terminal patient An incurably sick patient shortly before death (similar to Final-stage patient, Patient terminally ill).

Torah Teaching, Instruction. In its narrow sense it means the Pentateuch; in a wider sense it means the Hebrew bible and Talmud; in its widest sense it includes in addition all halakhic literature up to this day

Authors

Bleich, J. David, Rabbi, Herbert and Florence Tenzer Professor of Jewish Law and Ethics, Cardozo Law School, Yeshiva University, New York.

Bollag, David, Rabbi, Lecturer in Didactics of Jewish Religion at the College for Jewish Studies, Heidelberg; Lecturer at the Institute for Christian-Jewish Research at the University of Lucerne; Lecturer at the Dormition Abbey, Jerusalem.

Glick, Shimon, Director of the Lord Rabbi Immanuel Jakobovits Center of Jewish Medical Ethics, Professor and former Dean, Faculty of Medicine, Director of the Moshe Prywes Center for Medical Education, Soroka Hospital and Ben-Gurion University, Beer Sheva, Ombudsman for the Ministry of Health in Israel.

Goldschmidt, Lydia, R.N., M.A. Director of Nursing Division, Shaarei Zedek Medical Center; Lecturer on Ethics and Legal Aspects of Nursing, Henrietta Szold School of Nursing, Hebrew University Hadassah Medical School, Jerusalem.

Hitzig, Walter, Professor Emeritus of Pediatric Hemato-Oncology, Children's Hospital, University of Zurich. Former Vice President of the Central Ethic Committee of the Swiss Academy of Medical Sciences.

Hofstetter, Elias, Dr.iur., lawyer, former scientific assistant, Institute for Criminology, University of Bern.

Hurwitz, Peter Joel, M.D., Plastic and Reconstructive Surgeon, Project

Manager "Jewish Ethics and the Care of End-of-Life Patients,"
Institute for Jewish Studies, University of Basel.

Kravitz, Leonard S., Rabbi, Professor of Midrash and Homiletics,
Hebrew Union College, New York.

Küng, Hans, Professor Emeritus of Ecumenical Theology, University
of Tübingen.

Lamm Maurice, Rabbi and Professor, Chair in Professional Rabbin-
ics, Yeshiva University, New York; Founder and President,
National Institute for Jewish Hospice.

Marti, Mario, Lawyer and former scientific assistant, Faculty of Law,
University of Bern.

Picard, Jacques, Professor of General and Jewish History and Director
of the Institute for Jewish Studies, University of Basel.

Ravitsky, Vardit, Ph.D., Dept. of Philosophy, Bar-Ilan University,
Ramat Gan. Presently at Department of Clinical Bioethics,
National Institutes of Health, Bethesda, Maryland.

Steinberg, Avraham, Professor of Pediatric Neurology, Shaarei Zedek
Medical Center; Director of the Center for Bioethics, Hebrew
University Hadassah Medical School, Jerusalem; Head of
the Israel Governmental Committee concerning the Care
of End-of-Life Patients.

Index